Unhindered Childbirth

Wisdom for the Passage of Unassisted Birth

Sarah M. Haydock

SARAH HAYDOCK

ISBN:**1494949105**
ISBN-13:**978-1494949105**

"I want to do to you what spring does with the cherry trees."

~ Pablo Neruda

SARAH HAYDOCK

Contents

SARAH HAYDOCK

Preface

This book does not convey a narrow & rigid view of the way childbirth should be. It does not speak of one birth choice as higher than another, or of one choice as safer than another. Those are topics that could be argued to infinity without any real conclusion. Those sorts of arguments have no place in this book.

This book is about listening to your body's own wisdom and treading your own path; this book is about following your heart and discovering your own strength. This book is about my personal experiences with unassisted childbirth, and my passion for sharing this empowering journey with others. This is an inspirational resource and a guidebook, both for women who choose Unassisted Childbirth and for any women interested in blissful, pleasurable and joyous birth.

I know that for some, this book may be offensive. For some, it may raise concerns – it may seem frightening or radical. Of course for me, it is none of those things. For me, this book is about unearthing the experience of infinite passion and joy in the process of giving birth without interference. This book is about personal empowerment. It is about taking responsibility for your choices, learning to listen to your own body, and discovering your innate strength.

PART I:

Opening to Freebirth

Birth Happens

*"It's very rare to see an undisturbed birth in a modern U.S.
teaching hospital, but when you see a woman who isn't
frightened, who's giving birth without interference, you stand
back in awe and realize how little needed you are except in
the rare circumstance."*

~ Ina May Gaskin

Birth is the most powerful and beautiful event that I have ever experienced. It is a monumental happening and an enormous milestone in a mother's life, and yet, it is so, so simple. Birth carries such intensity – it can be earth-shattering... mind-blowing... orgasmic! And yet, birth is part of life as a whole, and no different from it. It is as effortless, as graceful and as natural as walking, singing, and sleeping. It may seem contradictory, but as much as there is nothing which resembles the power and intensity of giving birth, birth is equally a very simple process. Every human who has ever lived was born from their mother. Birth is both ordinary and extraordinary.

In mainstream culture and in the media, birth is often portrayed as something very complicated and painful. It requires complex instruments, precise measurements, and constant observation from professionals to ensure that the process progresses. I do not believe that birth requires *any* of this. Birth is a biological process like the beating of your heart – it happens, as all who have given birth naturally know well, without your "permission." It does not require you to *do* anything. In fact, in my experience, the more that you let go of trying to guide the birthing process, the more easily it flows.

All of my children were born without professional assistance. All of my birth experiences were uniquely ecstatic, empowering, and liberating. My experience tells me that birth is a completely natural process which requires no intervention, no observation, and no tools. Birth happens with or without your ideas or plans. Birth happens with or without professional guidance. Birth happens, and if you let it, birth can happen in unimaginable beauty and bliss.

My Story

My story starts just after my 21st birthday. I had never planned on becoming pregnant, but I met a man who swept me off my feet. I quit my job and spent nearly every moment with him. We swam naked in cold mountain streams, slept in the woods under a tarp, cooked over an open fire, made love in the rain... Every night we looked up at the stars together. I felt my wildness – my primal femininity – a part of me stirred that I never even knew existed. I was pregnant within a few months.

Since I had never really considered being pregnant, I had also never considered professional prenatal or birth care providers. The idea was totally foreign. I had never looked at a pregnancy book. Never spoken to anyone about pregnancy care. And so, naturally, I did not seek these things out. I felt comfortable being pregnant, and didn't even think to take additional steps. I suppose already in those days I had a sense of personal responsibility for my pregnancy and birth, not from a conscious choice, but out of my only awareness; my innate response to pregnancy was trust.

A few months in to that first pregnancy, people started to ask me what I planned to do – who I planned to "hire." When I answered, "nobody," I was told many frightening stories of death and pain and emergency childbirth situations that would be totally beyond my control, and I began to question my decision. I looked to books and stories. I read Veronika Robinson's and Ina May Gaskin's books. I read up on what happens in birth, and what to do if complications arise. I re-learned to trust, although my trust had been greatly shaken by those fearful stories. Would I die? Would it be unbearable? Would I be 'good' at giving birth?

When the night of the birth of my first child came, the fear left me completely. Slowly but surely the intensity grew, and my strength and capability became totally apparent. Peacy's birth was very powerful. She rocked me and pushed me into depths that I had never reached before. She showed me that I had nothing to fear – showed me the power that all women carry – showed me that birth is a rite of passage which flows, hidden, in our veins from the time we begin menstruating, through pregnancy, and into motherhood. Still, there was something missing from that birth which I could never put my finger on until after the birth of my second child.

Looking back, I can see that even though there were no birth professionals there with us in our little cabin, they were there in my head. The words and stories I had consumed during those last few moons of pregnancy stuck with me. I recall at one point, as Peacy was crowning, I felt pain. Out-of-body joy, but also great pain. Not knowing how to handle this, I remembered something Ina May Gaskin had written in her 'Guide to Childbirth,' and tried a bellow – an "animalistic" bellow as she had described, although, being forced, it was *anything* but primal. All it did, as I remember, was cause my body to tense up and was probably responsible for the bad vaginal tear I was left with after the birth. This goes to show that our own minds and beliefs are the real hindrance, even more so, maybe, than the physical presence of an unwanted birth attendant.

When I became pregnant again, I flipped through some books like I had in the last pregnancy, but got bored of that pretty quickly. It didn't seem necessary. I trusted this time, and the fear was gone, so why read if it wasn't enjoyable? Luckily at that time I lived without electricity, (and therefore, without an internet connection,) so I was not sucked into birth forums or caught up in searching for more birth stories online. As awesome as that is to do now that we live with electricity, I really do prefer the simpler and less electronic life. Without the stories and distractions, I was able to really just be with my body.

My pregnancy was rocky at first. Life in general was rocky. My partner was seriously ill, and I often wondered how much longer he would stay alive. I was anemic and exhausted, but after the first trimester, things looked up. Like my first pregnancy, this one was "unassisted," but there was a different level of trust this time.

When the night of Micah's birth came, I was so blessed! I learned much about myself, about inhibition, and about my ability to let go during that very short labor. At first I sat in the tub with a friend, but after a short time she left me alone in the bathroom – alone in the house. Just before she left, contractions had been mild. It felt like relatively early labor. Once she left, something shifted.

Knowing that I was alone – the total darkness – the complete safety and comfort of that space opened something in me – my primal, instinctual, animal nature was set *completely free*. Bars and chains that I did not even know existed melted away. My rational mind was gone. Contractions shook my body – tidal waves that sent me to my knees. I was super-human, a dark birthing goddess!! Micah was born in a few minutes. That night was the most transformative night of my life.

When I became pregnant for the third time, I learned that we never really reach an end in our journeys. I had always assumed that because Micah's birth was so blissful, and his pregnancy so full of trust, that my pregnancies and labors would always be that way from there on out. Not so. My third pregnancy was full of fear and doubt, and it took an incredible amount of strength and resolve to face that fear, and to come to terms with myself yet again. Ahmik's pregnancy and birth was yet again an enlightening passage; she taught me to let go of my stubborn desire to do things by myself; to graciously receive from others, and in doing so, to deepen my trust in humanity.

I feel so very lucky to have chosen "unassisted" birth from the start. I feel lucky for so many reasons; I never had to fight for my rights, to protect myself against invasion, to defend my privacy... I was free to birth in ecstasy and to experience those rights of passage in my own way, knowing from the beginning that I, and only I, was in charge. The main reason I feel grateful, however, is the powerful journey of personal discovery that these births brought me. Peacy's birth taught me that looking inward and trusting my own body is *always* a better idea than looking for advice from external sources. Micah's birth taught me that my greatest adversary in birth is my inhibition; his birth showed me a way to release that inhibition, and the results of that total release were so powerful. Ahmik's birth helped me to find my strength and let go of inhibition – to find true trust in the presence of another human.

Through these passages of pregnancy and birth, I have learned that childbearing autonomy is more than just making the choice not to hire a midwife. My journey to true autonomy is eternal. In my life, I am constantly peeling away layers of belief and conditioning which hold me back. I am constantly discovering deeper levels of myself, finding greater intimacy and ease. Pregnancy culminating in the intensity of birth is an incredible catalyst in this journey of self-discovery, a true and age-old rite of passage into greater self-awareness.

What's your plan?

A few weeks ago, I attended a small gathering of mothers and pregnant women. The gathering was dedicated to sharing our birth experiences, healing birth traumas, and welcoming the pregnant women into the world of motherhood. Some women present were pregnant for the first time. They had many questions about what to expect during childbirth.

One of the mothers at the gathering shared stories from the births of her six children. Even though many of her births took place in the same setting, they were all very different. Just as each child has an innate spark & presence, each birth carries its own unique energy.

We all start out with some sort of birth plan. Even if our plan is very loose, we all have some idea of what setting our birth might take place in and who might be there with us. Some women choose to birth in a hospital. Some choose to birth at home with a midwife. Some choose an unassisted birth. Some choose a planned cesarean. Some births go "as planned." Some don't.

The truth is, you can't really plan a birth. Birth happens in its own way – it flows through you like wind flowing through the leaves of a tree. It moves you, shakes you, rocks you, and largely it is a power beyond control.

Of course, you can plan the location of your birth, and you may find yourself there when labor begins, or make your way there shortly thereafter. Of course you can plan who might be there, and you may find them there at the birth, if they are not sleeping or sick or across the country or attending another birth. You can choose what you eat during pregnancy, and which herbs you steep in your tea, and the ways in which you nourish yourself, and these can certainly affect the birth process. But, essentially, the power of birth is not something you can plan for. When birth comes, it is like a spirit moving through you. The best thing you can do is to let go of your beliefs, plans, and ideas about birth and listen to that power in your body. The best thing you can do is to surrender to that earth-shaking power, and let it guide you.

Our beliefs about the way birth should look can limit our ability to experience birth in its full, raw beauty. Just as it would be difficult to experience real intimacy if we believed that love needed to look a certain way, so would it be difficult to experience the joy of birth if we believed that the birth process had to look a certain way. Having expectations is certainly helpful – that's whywe develop the habit of expecting certain things and planning ahead. (For example, it is helpful to expect that your baby will be exiting your body through your vagina. It is helpful to cook and freeze some meals ahead of time, so that you won't need to cook much for a few days after your baby's birth. It is helpful to know that your body is made to birth effortlessly. It is helpful to expect the unexpected.) Expecting birth to look and feel a certain way, however, can be and often is detrimental.

A few weeks ago, at that mother's gathering, the mother of six children finished telling her story. She looked over at the pregnant women who had asked what to expect in her first birth. "No two births are the same," she said.

Planning a birth is exciting and helpful, but getting stuck on that plan, if it is not where the birth energy is going, is a hindrance. Unhindered birth requires surrender.You can never know where your next birth will take you – you can never fully anticipate what the experience will be, for each woman is different, each child is different, and each moment is different.

Wherever you live in the world, I am sure you have seen leaves blowing in the wind. Here, near my home, the leaves of the Aspen trees are especially known for the way they shimmer and quake in the slightest breeze. These leaves do not resist the wind – they do not plan which way they will move next. They let the wind take them.

Just as the Aspen leaves quake in the wind, so birth moves us. Each birth carries its own power, and to experience it in ecstasy means surrendering to that unique power, whatever it may be.

Technicalities

What is unassisted birth? Because of the terminology, it is easy to look at unassisted birth and see something reckless – how can an 'unassisted' woman give birth safely? There are so many misconceptions around birth, and especially around unassisted birth.

I use this term "unassisted birth" because it has become a popular term in recent years. Unassisted birth does not mean birth without any assistance – it means birth without *professional* assistance.Unassisted birth does not necessitate solitary birth. Unassisted birth can be, and often is, social. Mostmodern humans choose to birth socially, but social birthing does not necessitate a midwife, doctor, or professionally trained birth attendant.

In traditional cultures, 'social birth' most often meant birth attended by some or many female family members. These family members were not professionally trained, but rather wise in the ways of their own bodies and instincts. These traditional birth attendants were there to support, encourage, and empower the birthing mother. Today, although our society is structured much differently than the societies of our tribal ancestors, "unassisted" births can come with powerfully supportive birth attendants. "Unassisted" birth can be assisted!

The real difference between unassisted birth and professionally-assisted birthis that unassisted birth comes "without the politics." Birth is not a medical event, and yet, in professionally-assisted births the political regulation put upon doctors and midwives forces birth to become medical, even when midwives or doctors have the best intentions. The rules surrounding these professional practices deny the possibility, in many cases, of a truly unhindered, truly free birth. That is why the term "freebirth" is also accurate, and I'll use the terms "unassisted birth" and "freebirth" interchangeably throughout this book.

There is a beautiful movement that I see in the works in our society – humans are waking up to the reality that self-reliance, (or communal-reliance,) has the potential to nourish, empower and sustain our lives in an infinitely greater way than reliance on political, medical, and economical systems. Freebirth is self-reliant birth.

Unhindered birth is a step beyond unassisted birth – a step beyond the freeing of our bodies from socio-political constraints surrounding childbirth. Unhindered birth means exploring, evaluating, and freeing ourselves from our *own*physical, mental and emotional constraints as well. Unhindered birth is simultaneously the epitome of freedom and the epitome of surrender. Unhindered birth means freeing yourself from all bondage, and *truly meeting yourself* in the throw of this major life event. This freedom and surrender in birth is a beautiful thing – a powerful, uncivilized, uncontrollable, unstoppable force that comes from *within*..

Why I Choose Freebirth

"All that is needed, all that is wanted at the time of birth is to be very quiet and on one's own. Yes, at this point you want to be by yourself because anything coming from the world outside truly intrudes. You have become so acutely sensitive that the slightest false note is like a stab. An unwanted question, people moving around carelessly, even a noise..."

~ "Letter from an Older Woman, Canada" from Frederick Leboyer's "Art of Giving Birth"

I have heard many beautifully intimate stories of women birthingwith midwives whom they have come to trust and love. I've also read stories of women birthing in ecstasy in hospitals, surrounded by a staff of total strangers. Hospital births and midwife-attended home-births can be pleasurable and joyous experiences, and are clearly the right choice for some women. My choice to birth without professional assistance is a personal one.

I fully support the role of midwife. There are so many beautiful, motherly, and inspiring women who call themselves midwives. Without them, I believe our culture would suffer. I fully support the well-meaning and respectful obstetrician, who, rather than controlling a woman during her birth experience, empowers her and helps her to realize her true potential. Although not always the case by any means, many women find that giving birth with a professional birth attendant present is not only helpful and inspiring, but also joyful.

I do not believe that any informed birth choice is better than another. Each woman knows what is right for her and her baby. I chose to give birth without professional assistance for personal reasons. I felt strongly that it was right for me, for my body, and for my infant children. It was and continues to be a choice that I feel deeply passionate about for myself, and here are a few reasons why:

1. It's Intimate & Safe:

> *"There is no moment in life when a woman is more physically and spiritually open than when her baby is crowning."*
>
> ~ *Veronika Sophia Robinson*

The first reason that I choose freebirth is simple: I prefer intimacy. I feel most comfortable by myself and with those I have grown to love as family. Birth is such an intimate moment that requires such surrender – such vulnerability – that the thought of strangers or mere acquaintances in my birthing space makes me feel very uncomfortable. I seem to be able to open fully, truly, and deeply when I am alone or with family, and for me, to birth in ecstasy absolutely requires this openness.

Of course "alone" is only a concept. We are never alone. When we are inside our homes, only walls separate us from the trees and plants that live just outside. There are always ants and spiders crawling around somewhere nearby. There are the spirits and ancestral memories that guide us, consciously or unconsciously. We are never alone. What I really mean is, I suppose, that I only open fully, not when I am alone, but when I feel completely safe. Intimacy requires safety.

To birth joyfully and openly, a feeling of full safety is essential. The human body is not designed to give birth in a state of fear. Fear puts the body in a primal state tension. We are prepared to run or to fight for our lives, whether we are conscious of it or not, and all other functions of the body are put on pause. Fear will stall the progress of a birth entirely, or slow it painfully. Birth in fear can be painfully traumatic.

There are just some humans who I personally do not feel fully safe with. There is something about the presence of strangers that puts me on guard, even if just slightly. They are uncharted territory. Then, there are the people who I will feel good and friendly with, until they say or do something unexpectedly that seems way out of line with my course in life. Then there are the people who I know in my heart I feel safe with – safe to be myself entirely, without anymoderation at all. Those people are rarer than I would like. Those are the only sort of people I would want at my birth.

Recognizing your honest experience is essential. Who do you feel safe with? Be true to your needs. I choose unassisted birth because it lets me choose who is present. It gives me full ability to tell people to leave if I need to be alone, without worry about their reaction.

The intimacy of my three births was incredibly welcome. I was able to draw myself inward and focus on the cues of my body, rather than what people were doing around me. Birth is a soft process. It requires flexibility, vulnerability, and suppleness. Tension and fear, which are often synonymous with one another, are antithetical to the birth process. Birthing "unassisted" let me be totally vulnerable. It let me drop all inhibition – it let me be "me" in all of my power, in all of my strangeness… it is intimate, like waking up and turning to make love with your partner before you even open your eyes… touch in the darkness, trust, awareness, warmth, gratitude… but nothing of fear.

2. It's Empowering!

*"Without our connections to each other and the earth,
without our mothers' wisdom, we forgot our power. When*

*we were told that we had no souls, no minds, and no sisters,
we believed it was true. When they told us that childbearing
was too dangerous and difficult for women, midwives, and
herbs, we believed it was true. But wise women live in our
dreams, our visions, our deepest memories. We hear their
whispers and we listen."*

~ Susun Weed

When I was around middle school age, I used to watch television…
A lot of television. I watched crime dramas and sitcoms, cartoons
and countless movies. At that point in my life, I was painfully cut off
from the beauty and the cycles of life. I did not know anyone who
was pregnant, and never really thought about the birth process. I
never really heard anyone speak much about birth, except when I
would hear the occasional comment from a classmate. ("Did you
know that having a baby is like trying to push a watermelon through
a hole the size of a lemon???")

It is such an interesting culture that we live in… Sometimes it is so
hard for me to understand how we got here, and why. I was lucky to
attend a really beautiful Waldorf school when I was growing up, with
amazing teachers, and still, despite all that, the mainstream culture
crept in. I used to watch a long-running TV show called 'Friends.'
I'm sure some of you know the show that I am talking about… In
one of the later seasons of Friends, the character named Rachel
becomes pregnant, and in the season finale, she gives birth to her
baby girl. I remember that episode so well. It was my introduction to
birth.

What I learned from that episode of Friends was that Birth is
painful. Birth involves being in a hospital gown on a hospital bed
under fluorescent lights, grunting and screaming as a team of doctors
and friends around you chants "PUSH! PUSH!" Then, you have your
baby, and she is taken to be tested. You are drugged and delirious,
and don't even really know what has just happened. This heartbreaking theme repeated itself in movies and other media images

throughout my early years, and so my view of birth was shaped.

I am so, so grateful that my birth experiences were not like this in reality. In fact, they were the opposite – they were intense, but they were calm. They were dark and naked and intimate. Above all, they were empowering.

When I was pregnant for the first time and planning an unassisted birth, I found stories, books and websites that inspired me. Despite an overwhelming energy of fear around the birth process coming from friends, family, and the culture as a whole, I was able to find resources that I trusted – mainly accounts of women who had birthed unassisted, and some informal statistics on the safety of unassisted birth. Through these resources, I overcame my fears of pain. I overcame my fears of death. I accepted responsibility for my body and my choice. I transformed my initial media-influenced view of birth, a narrow and confused image, into a powerful vision. I trusted myself, and I was ready to face the unknown, and I was excited.

I came away from each birth transformed. Once upon a time, I was meek. I was shy and quiet and submissive. I would never speak up for myself because I did not think I deserved to. Although I came to experience great beauty in the *world* in my later teenage years, I still had an image of *myself* as small, ugly, and delicate.

Birthing unassisted revealed to me that the awesome beauty and power, which I saw so clearly in the natural world, also resided in my own body. It showed me that women are the earth – we are strong, powerful, and so resilient. We are life-givers, and this power we hold is innate! It is not something that we need to be guided through – it is not something we must learn; our bodies are made to give birth, and what an amazing strength that is!

For those of you who have experienced the pure ecstasy that arises at the peak of your baby's crowning, as your baby bridges the space between your body and the outside world, as you are about to meet them and hold them and touch them to your breast, you know the power that I am referring to!

This power, for me, was amplified by the fact that, with the birth of my second child, there were no other humans present. My mate and my 21-month-old daughter were sleeping in a nearby cabin, and I was alone, in a different dwelling. It became so vivid & clear to me in that moment that I am strong – I am powerful. It became so clear that women - all women through the ages - have been and are dazzlingly, fiercely, and beautifully strong. Women are built to give birth – our bodies are designed to grow babies and bring them into the world. Birthing unassisted was a major turning point in my life, and the most empowering experience in my all my years on earth.

3. It'sTraditional:

> *"Women are carriers of life. We hold the fruit of our loving beneath our hearts. For too long we have lost touch with the fullness of this mystery due to modern, technological culture."*

> *~Jeannine Parvati Baker*

Today, what we call unassisted childbirth was once known simply as birth. It would be more accurate to call hospital & midwife-assisted births "assisted births," rather than labeling freebirth as the newcomer.

The word midwife, in many old languages and cultures, is synonymous with the word grandmother or wise woman. In tribal cultures, women who had given birth many times, and seen their daughters give birth, became these wise women. They attended the births of their grand-daughters to offer a token of support – as a symbol of the continuity of life. These women were family – they were not "certified grandmothers." They did not study in a school to learn how to support their granddaughters best. They knew through experience that they were present to support this young woman's journey – *not to guide her, but to inspire her.*

The modernization of birth is only the blink of an eye in human history. Birth has changed drastically in the past few hundred years. I believe it grew to be this way for two reasons: One clear and simple reason is that unassisted birth is not conducive to anyone making any money.

In this day and age, it seems as though everything is monetized to its highest potential. If you can convince someone that they need something to survive, then they will pay for it. When you convince a woman that she cannot birth without help from a professional, then there is money that stands to be made for that professional. A woman birthing alone or with her family does not have to pay anyone. In a society obsessed with money, unassisted birth does not fit in.

The second reason that I believe unassisted birth has fallen away from being the "norm" is more subtle. Unassisted birth is empowering to women and to the common family. It is harder to exert control over a person or a group if they are empowered – harder to keep a population in check if they know that they can care and provide for themselves. The fact that most people believe birth cannot function without professional assistance is beneficial to those who hold power in our society.

For all of human history, before medical birth became the norm, women were giving birth. Our ancestors gave birth with an innate trust that this was what they were built for. Their pelvises were clearly the right size. Their bodies would function. Why would a creature be designed to experience undue difficulty and hardship in birth? Wouldn't this put a damper on procreation?

> *"Anthropologists who've studied cultures where women were well-fed and watered, nurtured and cared for, have found no incidence of death in childbirth for such women. Humanity has been birthing unassisted since the beginning of evolution. If birth is the dangerous medical condition that we've been indoctrinated to believe, we simply wouldn't have survived as a species."*
>
> *~Veronika Sophia Robinson*

I choose freebirth because it is the way of my ancestors. However broken it may be, I choose to rejoin my tribe. However fractionated and distorted the ancient human in me has become, I still feel her. She is my true nature, and she will never leave me. Despite the confines of civilization, I am wild and free in my heart.

4. It's Liberating:

"You take your life in your own hands, and what happens?

A terrible thing: no one to blame."

~ Erica Jong

My birth experiences taught me that I am entirely capable of caring for myself. This does not mean that I shun advice or help from others. What it means is that I look to myself first, especially if I am experiencing frustration or difficulty. After giving birth without assistance, it became clear to me that I am so much more powerful than I ever could have imagined. My body and my spirit will guide me through life, and looking to external sources for healing and clarity is not always necessary. Most of the time, healing and clarity come from within.

Our culture does emphasize dependence on others for healing, learning, and fulfillment. We are told to seek love and joy everywhere but in our own hearts. We are told to seek miraculous cures for our health problems through drugs, doctors, and natural healers. Birthing without assistance was liberating for me – it revealed the innate power I have to create & change my own experience, without looking elsewhere.

This revelation is so inspiring. It does not mean that I do not depend on others. We are all interdependent. Life is an intricate and beautiful web, and no-one is alone or separate from it. Our personal human needs are closely intertwined with the needs of all humans, plants and animals living on this earth, as well as with the needs of earth herself... So no, I am not alone, but I am liberated ~ *I am*

22

liberated in my beliefs. I no longer believe myself to be a captive of any system. I no longer believe that I will find salvation in anything other than myself. I am my own teacher. I am my own healer. In this way, I take true responsibility for myself.

5. It's free (or can be):

When you choose unassisted birth, you don't need to pay to hire a care provider. Women and families often spend thousands of dollars on prenatal care and labor with each pregnancy, whether they opt for a hospital birth or a midwife. Insurance does cover some expenses, sometimes. It even covers midwife-assisted homebirths in some states. This is helpful, if you have insurance, but health insurance is costly as well.

The cost of a hospital birth can be upwards of $30,000. I have even heard of cases where the cost was closer to $200,000. Luckily, most women who choose hospital births have insurance, and often most of the costs associated with hospital births are covered by insurance.

The cost of home-birth varies. With CPM (certified professional midwife) homebirths or birth center births, the cost could be anywhere from $1,500 to $8,000. This usually includes a few prenatal visits, the labor, and a post-partum visit. Lay midwives usually charge less for their services, usually somewhere between $500 and $3,000. What insurance will cover in regards to a homebirth varies from state to state, and lay midwives are not likely to be covered by insurance.

Unassisted birth is free, or as free as you want it to be. Some women choose to rent a birth pool, or to invest in some plastic bed-liners to make cleanup easier. Some women choose to hire a post-partum doula to help with meals or care of older children after the birth. You really could assign any budget to freebirth, from absolutely free to extravagantly expensive.

At the time my first two children's births, I could have afforded to hire a midwife, but chose not in joy and excitement for the opportunity to birth without professional assistance. I feel that given my monetary means at those times, the fact that those UCs were extremely inexpensive was quite a valid advantage.

During my pregnancy, my costs were minimal. I invested in dried herbs and a few herbal tinctures to nourish me during pregnancy and to have on hand during labor. The total cost of these herbs was probably less than $75. I also bought a few books, and the total cost for those was probably around $50. I found a few of the books I was looking for through our small public library, which saved on cost. The second time around, I only bought a few bags of herbs – I had a lot left over from my first pregnancy! With my third pregnancy I chose to hire a doula on the off-chance that my two children, 3 and 4 years old at the time, were awake during my third child's birth. The cost of our doula was $600, but we never ended up calling her to come when I went into labor.

There are really no supplies that are essential during birth, apart from a warm space, a place to pee and poop, and your own body. As Veronika Sophia Robinson says, "Your tool kit is your body and your intuition." Supplies that might help, like towels and extra sheets, can often be found for free. In fact, I have some towels left over from my most recent birth that are looking for a new home as I write this.

6. It supports direct instinctual action:

This is the reason for choosing freebirth that I feel most passionate about. It is closest to my own heart, and the most applicable to experiencing an infinitely joyous birth. This last reason is directly related to the fluid energy that surges through a woman as she births her baby.

> *"The body is not the opposite of spirit. To feel spirit power is to be completely alive, and to do so we must fully inhabit our earthly bodies and our senses – not just sight, hearing, taste, smell, and touch, but also intuition {and} direct knowing."*
>
> *~Gail Faith Edwards*

When you choose unassisted childbirth, you choose to trust your own body and the processes of nature completely. You choose to be your own guide.

Birthing without professional assistance puts you in the center of the experience – you are the "expert," and you always have been. This leaves you physically, emotionally, and psychologically free to choose your location. To assume whatever position feels comfortable. To make love. To be totally naked. To do strange things because they feel right. To listen to your body.

Many midwives are happy to respect your power and freedom as a birthing mother – they understand that this is their duty as a birth professional. But I have read and heard so, so, so many sad stories of both doctors *and* midwives who took it upon themselves to direct the birth of their clients without their client's expressed call for assistance. This takes the form of asking thebirthing women to assume different positions, asking her to lie down to have her progress checked, telling her that labor is not progressing quickly enough, or insisting that mechanical intervention is necessary. Some women describe being drugged without permission, having their waters broken without permission, or being told against their better judgment that some sort of intervention was necessary.

This kind of intervention is highly detrimental to the birthing woman. It interrupts, hinders, and even reverses the flow of the birth energy and the progression of labor. When a doctor tells a woman that her labor is taking too long, it is a self-fulfilling prophecy. It causes stress, which in turn makes the labor take even longer. One intervention leads to the next. What we really need while we birth our babies is to be left alone. Interventions should *only* ever take place when there is a clear request for help from the mother.

I cannot imagine having the routine procedures of a medical birth asked of me during the intensity of labor. Birth required every ounce of my attention. It required that I was fully present in my body and listening entirely to its cues. To be pulled back into someone else's views and expectations of birth would be antithetical to the process itself.

In too many cases, even worse situations are described in which doctors and midwives act and make choices that involve a birthing woman's body against her overtly expressed will. This is rape. It is traumatic and devastating, not only to mothers who suffer the emotional and physical damage, but also to entire families. When a woman's body is penetrated with human hands or machines, despite her verbal or physical resistance, it is an attack …an assault. Her autonomy is taken. In a time as intense and vulnerable as birth, this can be highly confusing, especially if it is being verbally justified by the doctor or midwife.

When I hear stories of birth rape, my heart grows heavy. I question how humanity ever reached this barbaric and perverse point. Women should not need to fight for their autonomy at a time as intense and vulnerable as birth. These actions are a breach of human rights, and should not be allowed in any way, shape or form. These acts are acts of overt violence. If you do not choose unassisted birth, then make sure to get to know your birth care-provider very well. Make sure you are clearly heard and respected, and that you trust them fully. Maybe even more importantly, make sure that *they trust you*.Without trust and respect on both ends, the natural flow of birth will not be able to occur.

> *"Undisturbed birth represents the smoothest hormonal orchestration of the birth process, and therefore the easiest transition possible; physiologically, hormonally, psychologically, and emotionally, from pregnancy and birth to new motherhood and lactation, for each woman. When a mother's hormonal orchestration is undisturbed, her baby's safety is also enhanced, not only during labor and delivery, but also in the critical postnatal transition from womb to world."*

~*Sarah Buckley*

For me, unassisted birth provided a safe space in which no-one's will, however harmless or well-intentioned their will might have been, was ever imposed upon me. No one ever asked me to lie down so they could check my progress. No one ever suggested a different position, or asked me to tell them what I was experiencing. I was free to follow my own body's cues.

When you listen to your body, (which it is actually hard *not* to do during labor if you are left unhindered,) birth flows so effortlessly. Choosing freebirth let me act immediately on each impulse as it arose. If I had an impulse to gently shake my belly, I did it. If I had an impulse to change position, or make a certain sound, or drink water or eat, I did. If I wanted to be in the bath or get out of the bath, I did. If I wanted to do things that made absolutely no sense at all, I did them. Often, something that makes no sense at all is really a cue from your baby that s/he needs something from you, and who knows – maybe that need is crucial.

Later in this book, I will share the birth stories of my three children. I believe that the ecstasy of their births was due to my immediate action on each impulse as it arose. In birth, there is sometimes no time to question why something feels right. If you wait – if you stop to question your intuition & your impulses, then great unnecessary discomfort or pain can ensue. Discomfort and pain are not inherently bad, but undue pain is nothing that anyone needs during birth. When you trust your own body's (and your baby's) wisdom and let them guide you, birth can become blissful. For me, unassisted birth was the perfect way to ensure that this would be the case.

When to Choose (& when Not to Choose) Freebirth

This chapter is really very simple. Choose an unassisted birth when your heart opens wide at the prospect. Choose an unassisted birth when it is your clear choice *for you* – not when it is what someone else chooses for you or for them. Every woman knows what is best for her body, and for her baby. Listen to your intuition, and to your heart. Find that place of deep knowing within yourself, and make your choice from there.

I often hear people say that they support unassisted birth for "low risk women." If you've been told that you are "high risk" but you don't believe it – if you trust in your body to birth without professional assistance, then listen to your heart. Tread the path that you wish to tread, and know your strength. If you've been told that you are "low risk" but you just feel deeply that you'll want some support from a professional, than listen to those deep feelings.

For me, I always knew that unassisted birth was my choice. I questioned it at times, especially with my third pregnancy, but always found clarity within. Listen to your body. Listen to your baby. Listen to your intuition, and make your choice accordingly. Remember also, just because you choose something does not mean that it has to remain your choice. Things always change in unexpected ways, and there's no need to hold on to an outdated choice just because you spent a lot of time or energy making it

PART II:

Pregnancy & Preparation for Birth

"Nature does not hurry, yet everything is accomplished."

~ Lao Tzu

Pregnancy is such a beautiful passage. From the moment of conception until you birth your baby's placenta, you and your baby are joined. Your body is your baby's world – a soft pink cocoon full of muffled sounds and the ever-beating "thump... thump..." of your heart's rhythmic pulse. When I was pregnant for the first time, I felt more than ever like my body was an image of the fertile earth, and my womb the ocean, full of the deep mystery of life.

Pregnancy is a time of growth and nourishment, not only for your growing baby, but also for you as a woman. Pregnancy is the bridge between womanhood and motherhood – a space in which to grow and to nurture yourself – to learn to listen to your body and trust your instincts. Pregnancy is a time to face your fear. If you have never given birth before, you are coming up against the unknown, and for some this can feel terrifying.

Know that fear is natural, and when it is not avoided or ignored, fear can be transformed. When faced, fear can come full circle – it can become a deep trust and a deep inner knowing that you are a powerful woman with the strength and grace to birth your baby. Fear can become confidence, faith, excitement and conviction.

Here in this chapter, I will share ways of nourishing and caring for yourself, not only through foods, herbs, rest and bodily movement, but also through emotional and spiritual empowerment, bodily awareness, and learning to face and let go of outdated beliefs and fears. From the moment your baby is conceived, you are her nourishment. The food you eat, the sounds you make, your sleep, your movements, and your love all feed her. Pregnancy presents an amazing opportunity to learn how to truly nurture yourself, and in doing so, to create a deeply nourishing prenatal world for your baby.

Prenatal Care

*"A small percentage of couples and single mothers choose to
provide their own prenatal care, paying close attention to a
lifestyle that supports a healthy pregnancy… These women
recognize that excellent self-care and intuitive awareness can
guide them through pregnancy and birth safely, joyously, and
in optimal health. This is a very empowering experience and
creates a deeply intimate atmosphere in the family. In my
own family, we have had three such pregnancy experiences…
I have found that by looking inward for the information
about my wellness and my baby's health, I have developed
an enduring confidence in my body, as well as deep
connections with my children. One need not be a midwife to
achieve this level of awareness."*

~Aviva Jill Romm, M.D. & Midwife

Choosing to have an unassisted birth does not necessarily mean
an unassisted prenatal period. Prenatal visits with a midwife are
often merely a visit from a nurturing mother-figure —a time for
relaxation, birth talk, laughter, belly massage & welcome support – a
time to voice fears, gain confidence and let things flow. Other times,
these visits may involve routine testing and examination. Remember

that it's always your choice whether you feel you need a test done or not.

There are many options to choose from when it comes to professional prenatal care. Many care providers don't necessarily care if you are planning to have an unassisted birth. They are happy to see you once or twice, or even for your whole pregnancy, without any sort of commitment on your part. Some, however, will not wish to see you during your prenatal period if you do not plan to sign on for the whole pregnancy and birth. It depends largely on the legal restrictions of your state.

I understand where they are coming from. Our society is quite complicated. Who would want to have their license to practice revoked over something that happened during the birth process of one of their clients, even if they were not at all involved in the birth itself? They want to have a degree of control over the situation, and only work with clients that agree with their view of the way birth needs to happen safely. Even Ina May Gaskin, a pioneer in the homebirth movement, makes mention of this in her book *Spiritual Midwifery*. She warns her audience of aspiring midwives to be wary of a woman who does not give pre-labor consent to be transported to the hospital if necessary, saying such women are too high risk to be served by a midwife in a home birth. Who is to blame her... Midwives and doctors accept some degree of responsibility for the wellbeing of their patients, which makes them legally vulnerable.

In that regard, if you are planning an unassisted birth but would like to have professional prenatal care, make sure you find a provider who is aware of your choice and supports it wholly. (Otherwise, you can always inform your provider that the baby came so quickly that you just didn't have any time to call.)

I chose not to seek professional prenatal care during my first twopregnancies. I trusted my body and the natural process of pregnancy and birth, and although it may have been enjoyable, professional prenatal care didn't seem necessary. My partner and I were my caregivers, and it was a very beautiful experience. I learned to trust myself. I learned to recognize when things did not feel right, and took action when necessary through lifestyle changes and herbal remedies. I learned to listen to my body and nourish my whole being. This self-care gave me a very strong prenatal connection with both my children, and even more so, it gave me a strong confidence in my ability to give birth.

I was more stressed during the first few months of my third pregnancy than I had been with my first two. I didn't feel as able to be my solo care provider, nor did I feel as connected with this baby as I had with my first two, and so during the end of my second trimester I sought prenatal care. I'm sure I *could* have continued to be my own support, but I was struggling emotionally with the idea of integrating a third child into our home, and the support, which came in the form of a visit with a midwife, was incredibly welcome. Although talking through my stress with Joey was helpful, what I really needed was another woman, someone with experience, to voice my fears, doubts, pains and thoughts to. She was strong, wise, and fully supportive of my choice to birth without professional assistance. One visit with her was all I needed to feel revitalized in my ability to care for myself and connect with my baby.

Learning to Listen to your Body (& Your Baby)

*"Looking within, listening within, rather than outside
ourselves is the key to a flowing birth. It is this moving
within, rediscovering our intuition, that shows us our
power."*

~Veronika Sophia Robinson

Receptivity to the needs of your body and your baby is of the utmost importance when you are giving birth. As you and your baby are rocked by the birth dance, you will feel urges and impulses to move, to sway, to moan, to rest, to drink water, to be warmer, colder, in a different location, or to do any number of strange and seemingly meaningless things. You may feel the need to be touched, or the need to be alone. You might feel called to speak something aloud, or you might want others to stop speaking. Whatever the impulse is, it is so essential to recognize that impulse and act on it as soon as you recognize it.

Ideally, while you are giving birth, there will be no barrier between the arousal of an impulse and your action upon it.

If birth follows its natural course, it flows like a river flowing to the sea, without interruption. When there is hesitation or fear of acting on an impulse, this creates a dam in that river. The water pools before the dam, and pressure builds there. It is impossible to stop the flow of the water; the river will find its way to the sea, but the dam will hinder the natural flow. When you act without hesitation on your impulses, this lets the river of birth flow naturally, and unobstructed.

Learning to recognize these impulses is the process of learning to perceive your intuitive voice. It is the process of re-learning to trust those seemingly insignificant feelings, sensations, images, and other subtle (or often not so subtle) sensitivities that arise in you on a daily basis. Oftentimes it is more difficult than you would think to recognize what is truly happening for you. A certain sensitivity is often layered upon by years of social conditioning, and digging through those layers may seem frightening, or may even be met with full-on resistance from your ego.

The following is an example of how social conditioning can affects us during birth:

You may have been told as a child that it is rude to tell someone to leave your home – after all they are a guest. You may have been told by your teacher not to say something that could hurt someone's feelings. I remember being told, over and over as a child, "*if you don't have anything nice to say, don't say anything at all.*" Even if these comments were said in passing and in a certain context, your younger self's brain may have internalized it and set it as a mode of operation – a way to survive and successfully navigate your life.

Fast-forward ten, twenty or thirty years. You are giving birth, unassisted, in your home with only your husband there. Deep down, something is off. Birth is not progressing and you don't know why. You may feel uncomfortable with his presence, but it may be hard to recognize this feeling due to all of the layers of thought that get piled upon it. (This person is my life partner... I love him... I wanted him here... He has always supported me... He deserves to be here, even if it is uncomfortable for me... It is his baby too... I am uncomfortable because there is something wrong with me... Asking him to leave the room would be unkind and rude... He will be upset with me... and so on.) So, so, so many layers of thought. Digging through these layers is tedious and creates a tremendous barrier between your intuitive voice, which clearly says "ask them to leave, even if just for a minute" and the social conditioning, which says, "no matter what, don't hurt somebody's feelings." After all these layers suppress the initial impulse, it is sometimes difficult to find it again. In everyday life, this manifests as a small problem – a bit of tension or a bad mood, until you express what you need to express. In birth, this can manifest at a whole new level – it can cause labor to become painfully slow or just plain painful. It can make you feel hopeless, immobilized, and cut off from your power.

> *"There is no agony like bearing an untold story inside of you."*
>
> *~ Maya Angelou*

Each and every experience we have, including physical sensation, emotion, thought and intuition, is important to recognize. We are not built of parts – we are whole, and learning to feel and experience ourselves as whole is the first step.

"The concept of being body-centered does not mean to imply separation of the body, mind, and emotions. In fact, all of these faculties are inextricably connected and interwoven in the organism we call human... However, it is possible for your thoughts to subvert your emotions and physical sensations in a culture where we are taught to do so. Being body-centered means unlearning the process of subverting your body, while still using your intelligence."

~ Aviva Jill Romm

It may sound complicated, but in fact, learning to listen to yourself – to your physical senses, your thoughts, your feelings, and your intuitive voice – as one whole being is quite simple. You naturally do it already. Your body tells you when it is time to eat or to sleep. Your soul calls out to you when it is tired of being alone – when it wants to connect with another being. You are drawn to certain places as you walk in a forest, or a field, or a park. You know when you need to pee. Your whole self has an innate intelligence, and it is constantly at work. It is helpful, when preparing for birth, to get to know yourself – to recognize these sensations as they arise and act upon them, and notice how much more smoothly life flows when your needs are not subverted by social conditioning.

Pregnancy is an amazing time to practice this. For one thing, your body, emotions, and intuition are extra-attuned during this time. Your dreams are often vivid. Your sense of smell is heightened. For another, all the changes you are going through at this time make these impulses easy to recognize due to the simple fact that they are different from the impulses of your non-pregnant self; foods that you once loved may taste repulsive to you all the sudden, and foods you never thought about may call out to you. Lastly, your baby gives you clear physical cues all the time throughout the day, be it through playful movements, peaceful stillness, or agitated kicks. Only you can know what your baby's movements mean.

When my daughter was inside of me, she would kick me if I sat still for too long. She wanted me to move around, so that she could find a different position that was more comfortable, or, maybe she was just bored. All I know is, I had the impulse to move when she kicked me, and once I was moving around again, she seemed to settle in to peaceful sleep. She needed the stimulation & movement to feel comfortable, I think. (Even now as a five-year old, she still needs it.)

Distinguishing between the impulses that arise spontaneously and the ones that arise out of social conditioning is helpful. Once you have gained an awareness of your experience, try to distinguish between what is socially conditioned and what is primal. Primal impulses are the only ones that have any place when you are giving birth.

Birth is not civilized. It does not follow anyone's law. It does not wait its turn. It is not polite or reserved. Birth is primal. Birth has a natural course, and follows that course whether you are ready or not. Trying to tame it, or to tame yourself while you are in its power, is always wasted effort. Learn to let go. Learn to surrender. Learn to free yourself of social conditioning. Learn to trust your instincts and your body. You are infinitely beautiful. You are worth it. You deserve the best that *you* have to offer yourself.

During pregnancy, learn to recognize and be honest with yourself about the self-criticism & doubt that arises in any situation. Notice when something is on the tip of your tongue, but you hold it inside out of fear. Notice if you choose not to eat, even when you're hungry, or choose not to sleep even though you're exhausted. Notice what you say to yourself when you see your reflection in the mirror. Notice what you do in an effort to please others, despite your own needs.

Do not try to suppress these things at first – let them happen. Notice them for what they are: social conditioning. Notice what sort of situations trigger them. Once you are aware of this, you can start to practice letting this conditioning go and acting on the original impulse. If you are hungry & notice a habit of denying yourself food, notice that habit. Let it go, and eat. If you're exhausted but feel compelled to wash the dishes because you know your husband is coming home soon, really notice this. Let it go, and rest. If you feel the need to say something but hold your tongue in fear of rejection, really notice this. Let the fear go, and speak.

The more often we act on our original impulses, the easier it becomes. Pregnancy is such a perfect time to notice any fragments of outdated beliefs that may trouble us, whether it is that we must always be polite, or that we must put others needs first, or that we must appear physically graceful & composed. These beliefs have no place in our bodies during birth.

When we establish new self-loving habits in the place of the old negative habits before giving birth, it makes the whole process easier. When we learn to trust our intuition and have the self-confidence to act upon it without fear, birth is allowed to flow. It flows naturally, beautifully, blissfully – unobstructed, and untamed. When you learn to trust your instincts, you learn to surrender to that ancestral power rushing through you.

Immersion in Nature

"We need the tonic of the wilderness."

~Henry David Thoreau

*"I encourage you to retrace the threads of your sacred
relationship to the earth. They are deeply encoded within
you.... If you stay with a place long enough, the land itself
will begin to teach you.... Personal growth depends on our
ability... to remember our true nature... our ability to open
our wild hearts in love and resonance with all of nature."*

~Gail Faith Edwards

There is nothing as opening, freeing, and grounding as spending time in the natural world. The earth and all her children are intertwined, interconnected, and fully animate. Each tree has its own breath. Each flower shines with its own light. The earth herself has a living, ever-beating pulse. If we learn to open ourselves to nature, to see her in her unbroken beauty, she has so much to offer us in return!

We are not separate from nature. We are a part of her, and we are as entwined in her cyclical beauty as we let ourselves become. It is impossible to avoid or to ever be truly cut off from the beings that live around us. The vast and intricate web of interconnection binds us together. Each time our foot touches the ground, we change the structure of the soil there. Each breath we take is made up of the exhalation of an infinite number of trees and plants. We leave a little of ourselves behind wherever we go, and in each moment, we are taking in a little bit of everything around us.

Recognizing that nature is our true origin gives us a sense of place – a sense of understanding and kinship. It shows us our own innate power, for when we truly see the majesty of nature and know ourselves to be a part of her, we see ourselves as bearing that same majestic strength and power.

Through relation to all of nature, the power of the feminine becomes so evident.

During pregnancy, taking the time to be in nature is so healing and empowering. It has amazing benefits for your physical, emotional & spiritual well-being. Being close to nature has proven time and time again to help heal many health conditions, including cardiovascular and respiratory problems as well as anxiety and depression.

Listening to the wisdom of nature gives us trust in our bodies. Seeing the effortless life cycles of the trees and the plants and other animals – recognizing the innate wisdom they carry through their lives – offers us confidence in our inborn ability to give birth. Our bodies are part of these effortless cycles. The wisdom inerrant in procreation is inherent in us – this ancestral knowledge is encoded in our cellular memory. It is not something that must be learned.

Wherever you may live, connection with nature is always possible. Most of my life I have lived in places where all I had to do was step out my front door to feel the churning life-energy of nature. I have lived briefly in small cities, too, where walking a bit was necessary to find that energy. Even if you live in a larger city, surrounded by concrete, you would be hard pressed not to find a little seedling poking up through a crack in the sidewalk, or a tree growing wild in the sparse soil by a friend's home. Sometimes, the natural beings who inhabit cities are the strongest teachers. They find a way to grow and spread, even in the harshest of environments. They have so much wisdom to offer.

When we as humans are inside buildings for long periods of time, the walls around us start to create not only physical barriers, but also emotional and spiritual barriers to the natural world. Often without noticing, our sense of connection can start to fade, and its place can be taken by mundane domestic worries or hyper-focus on the details of our civilized lives. Too often in our culture, we find ourselves inside houses, cars and shops all day long, only spending short periods of time outside. I find that when I deliberately set aside time to take a walk away from my civilized life, even if I feel there is too much to do, my whole day is brightened. As Henry David Thoreau once wrote, "an early morning walk is a blessing for the whole day."

Fresh air and immersion in nature is your best remedy, and your best prenatal care. Take walks by yourself. Go as far into the natural world as your legs will take you. Sit with a tree, or a flower, and listen to what she has to say. Let nature be the soil in which you spread your human roots. Let her nourish you, body and soul.

Nutrition

Food provides our bodies with a source of vital life-energy. Not long ago in human history, food was the foundation of society. Meals were eaten communally, and there was a shared gratitude and joy for the chance to share in the nourishment given by the food. Although our daily lives differ greatly today from the lives of our ancestors, that fundamental human necessity for nutrition remains the same.

During pregnancy, nutrition is central to the health of you and your baby. Well-nourished mothers have an easier time birthing, breastfeeding, and caring for their babies, while poorly nourished mothers can have complications during pregnancy, birth, and breastfeeding. During pregnancy, a nutritious diet can help to ease many common pregnancy ailments including nausea, anemia, constipation, bloating and fatigue.

It takes a great deal of energy to grow your baby. As Susun Weed says, *"During pregnancy, you create the cells needed to form two extra pounds of uterine muscle, the nerves, bones, organs, muscles, glands, and skin of your fetus, several pounds of amniotic fluid, a placenta, and a fifty percent increase in your blood volume!"* Nourishing your pregnant body and supplying your baby with the energy she needs is an amazing undertaking, and one that is greatly supported by eating a diet that is nutrient rich, calorie dense, appealing, and filled of the simple joy of food.

"Wise women see that most of the problems of pregnancy can be prevented by attention to nutrition. Morning sickness and mood swings are connected to low blood sugar; backaches, hypertension and severe labor pains often result from insufficient calcium…. Pre-eclampsia, the most severe problem of pregnancy, is a form of acute malnutrition."

~Susun Weed

Learning to eat well during pregnancy is about learning to love and listen to your body. Your body knows what it needs – it has an innate intelligence which guides you to the foods that would be most nourishing. Stock your kitchen with nutritious foods and your body will know which of these foods it needs – your body & your baby will tell you when you've had enough kale, or enough chicken, or enough sweet potatoes. It will tell you what is missing from your diet through cravings. *Learn to listen to what your body is telling you. Really.*

Learning to eat well is about learning to let go of your ideas of what you *should* eat when those foods don't work for you, and eating the nutritious foods that you love. It is about recognizing when you are hungry and what you are hungry for. It is about cherishing mealtimes as a time to care for, nourish, and support your growing baby, and it's about developing a loving and joyous relationship to food.

To obtain optimal nourishment through food, love and gratitude for the food we eat is so important, and just as important is our ability to let go of stress and anxiety around food. Often, it seems we get hung up on the nutritional value or the caloric intake of food we eat, and forget entirely to enjoy our food. When we lose the joy of eating, our food ceases to nourish us.

Eating well during pregnancy is not just about eating a certain number of calories a day, or making sure to obtain the "recommended dietary allowance" of every vitamin and mineral necessary for a healthy pregnancy. It is not about eating *"2 servings of whole grains and 3 servings of orange vegetables and 4 servings of protein and…..."* Trying to count and manage your food takes all the joy out of eating! It can drive you crazy, and it can also harm your digestive system. I know from experience.

Let me share a story from my first pregnancy that illustrates this point:

When I was in the final trimester of my first pregnancy, my skin started to feel itchy. It was a cold winter, and we were running our woodstove 24/7 to keep warm, so I thought maybe it was just due to dry skin from the cold weather and the woodstove. Then it got worse. My arms and legs, my hands and feet, my belly… then my whole body was unbearably itchy! It was worse after meals and before bed.

I knew something was wrong, and through some research I found that I was probably experiencing a liver ailment specific to pregnancy. My liver was incredibly stressed and could no longer properly process the foods that I was eating or the hormones that my body was secreting, and in turn was attempting to release toxins through my skin, causing it to itch. Once I learned this, I made some immediate diet changes and started making daily teas of liver-supporting herbs like dandelion, milk thistle, yellow dock, and burdock. This seemed to help immensely with the itchiness.

When I became pregnant again a year later, I waited to see what would happen. Some sources claim that if you experience this liver problem once, then you're very likely to experience it in subsequent pregnancies. Thankfully, I didn't experience any liver problems the second time around.

Why this happened, no one will ever really know, but I have a pretty strong inkling. I believe this liver disorder was caused by my eating what I thought I was supposed to eat during that first pregnancy, rather than what my body was actually asking for. I had it all figured out: two servings of orange veggies, 80 to 100 grams of protein a day, lots of whole grains, however much vitamin C…. I made it all fit in, every day, whether I was hungry for it or not, because I thought I was doing what was best for my baby and me.

I wasn't listening to my body. I overloaded myself with foods that I wasn't really hungry for, and deprived myself of the foods that I craved. I had ideas of what foods were "good" for me and what foods were "bad." At the time, I was extremely influenced by Sally Fallon and the "nourishing traditions" diet. I didn't even let myself eat ice cream more than a few times during that pregnancy because of the sugar content.... and I love ice cream!

This overload of foods that my body wasn't asking for caused a huge stress on my digestive system and my liver. It took a few months for my digestive system to recover after I gave birth to my daughter.

A shaky digestive system not only compromises your physical well-being, but also your body's energy levels and your emotional well-being. This, coupled with the added stress of a newborn, made those first few months after I gave birth very difficult.

When I became pregnant again, I had at least partially learned my lesson. This time, I ate what I wanted, when I wanted, without worrying that I wasn't eating enough or that I wasn't eating the right foods. I still ate a diet of unprocessed and organic food, but I didn't count grams and calories and servings this time around. I let my body be my guide, and felt much better in doing so.

During my third pregnancy, I was able to let go of my stress around food even more, and even included plenty of white (processed, oh no!!) rice, ice cream, and lots and lots of unprocessed sugar and chocolate. I even drank coffee a few times, but found that my body really rejected it, and I felt extremely nauseous afterwards.

This is all a very long story with a very simple moral: Don't let anyone tell you what is good for your body if it doesn't feel good – don't force something upon yourself because you've heard that it is "healthy" or necessary. No food is "healthy." Food is either nutritious or not. Eating nutritious food is second-nature. Ice cream? Nutritious. Kale? Nutritious. Butter? Nutritious. Unprocessed sugar? Nutritious! Learn to listen to your body's messages. Let your intuition guide you when it comes to food, and you'll probably feel much better, and happier!

"Be open to your needs and don't get stuck on any preconceived idea."

~*Aviva Jill Romm*

Don't get too caught up in a pregnancy diet.

If you crave scalloped potatoes with tons of real butter and real cheese, then eat scalloped potatoes, even if you call yourself a vegan, and enjoy every last bite! If you can't stand the thought of beef liver, then for the love of god don't force it upon yourself just because you think it's healthy! Nourish yourself with good ice cream and dark chocolate, if that is what you truly crave. Eat cookies when you want cookies. Find ways to make your food as high in nutrients as possible, but if you really crave white rice, which has a low nutrient value, then don't stress – maybe sometimes your body just needs energy more than it needs nutrients.

Every woman has unique dietary needs, and only she can know what these are through experience. The key to optimal nutrition during pregnancy is to follow your intuition.

If it rings true for you,be as close to your food as possible. Wild foods are always potent and nourishing. Gather wild dandelion leaves, nettles, raspberries, and any other foods that might grow wild near you if you can identify them and the season is right. Avoid wild foods that grow by roadsides or train tracks – look in woodlands and fields. Wild game, like venison & duck, is also very nourishing.

Food you grow yourself is also very potent, and the connection with your food that you get from raising it yourself is such a blessing. If you would enjoy doing so, grow a garden or raise chickens for eggs or meat.

You can also find closeness to your food by going to local farmers markets, or directly to farms, and developing relationships with the people who produce your food.

When buying from the store, if you can afford organic, pesticide-free produce, then aim to eat mostly organic.These foods do come at a higher price though, so if you cannot afford them, then enjoy what you can afford, knowing that your love of food is more important than whether or not it is organic.

Salt is good. Real sea salt contains tons of trace minerals, including magnesium, which support overall health and vitality, prevent high blood pressure, and prevent water retention during pregnancy. Use unprocessed salt from the sea, or unprocessed naturally mined salt. Don't use "table salt" if possible. Table salt is highly processed and contains toxic additives.

Don't be afraid of fat and sugar. Fats and sugars, when unprocessed, are highly nutritious. Rapadura or 'Sucanat' are two forms of unprocessed cane sugar that are very high in iron and other minerals. Maple syrup is also very nutritious. Sugar is not bad for you. Fats, like butter, coconut oil, etc., are essential! Many vitamins are not able to be absorbed unless couple with fat – these are called "fat soluble vitamins." Without fats, your body will not be able to absorb these!

Here are some of my thoughts on grains: "White" grains, like white rice and white flour, have gotten a pretty bad name in the 'health food' world. It is true that they don't contain much in the way of nutrition – basically they just contain a large energy boost. But sometimes, what our body really needs is energy! My personal opinion is that coupled with a nutritious diet, "white" grains are not going to hurt you. Whole grains can be extremely hard to digest, for some. I ruined my digestive system by thinking I had to replace allrefined grains with whole grains, and since letting go of that idea and including some white rice in my diet rather than brown rice, and using white flour is some of my baking and bread-making, my digestion has greatly improved. (If whole grains are what you really love and you digest them well, then of course you should eat them as much as you want. Everyone is different.)

Here are my thoughts on dairy: Milk is highly nutritious. It works well for me, but not everyone. Grass-fed cows produce milk that is more nutritious than grain-fed cows. If you like drinking milk, see if you can find a local farmer who sells raw milk. Grass-fed raw milk has amazing benefits for your digestive system!

And did you know that chocolate it nutritious? And coffee? And bacon? And eggs? So many of the foods that have been labeled "unhealthy" are actually highly nutritious foods. The main thing is to listed to your body – eat what feels right to you. Love your food. Love your body. Love nourishing your baby, and love yourself.

Herbal Nourishment during Pregnancy

*"Wise women know that we are each whole and unique, in
an individual, ever-changing, symbolic relationship with
herbs. Wise woman healing is grounded, earthed, rooted..."*

~Susun Weed

Cultivating relationships with the healing herbs that grow around us can enhance the vibrancy of life in so many ways. In a culture that emphasizes dependence on others for healing, these healing plants can help us to realize our innate freedom. Taking the time to acquire a bit of herbal wisdom can foster both physical and emotional well-being.

It was during pregnancy that I first began to develop a deeper relationship to the healing powers of herbs. All of my life, plants have fascinated me. As a child I remember exploring the plants that grew near my home. As I grew, I began to know them... to learn from them. I learned about growth, perseverance, relationship, beauty, death, and the cyclical nature of life. I learned that these plants could bring me immense joy.

When I became pregnant, however, it suddenly dawned on me that there was so much more to be learned from these plants. Apart from being incredible teachers and guides, herbs can nourish, tone, and restore balance our physical bodies. During pregnancy, herbs can help us to nourish our babies and ourselves. They can help us to overcome physical barriers like exhaustion, nausea, anemia, digestive problems, internal organ imbalances, skin problems, and infections.

> *"There is no great secret to good health. Despite the*
> *bombardment of advertisements from the health and beauty*
> *industries that offer an instant pill or cure-all for the woes*
> *and illnesses of life, good health is, in truth, the practice of*
> *living healthfully every day."*
>
> *~ Rosemary Gladstar*

Herbs are not like pills which will solve all your problems when you let yourself become unhealthy. They are not drugs. They are not replacements for a healthy lifestyle. Herbs provide nourishment for your body and soul, so that you will shine more vibrantly than ever. As Rosemary Gladstar says, "don't wait until you're sick to use herbs. The best way to cure illness is not to become ill, and there is a wonderful variety of longevity, nutritive, and tonic herbs that can and should be used daily to enhance wellness."

In this chapter, I will share with you traditional ways of preparing herbs, as well as the specific herbs and herbal remedies that I've found helpful in my personal pregnancy experiences. I'll also share pregnancy herbs that I haven't used personally, but which come highly reputed by herbalists and midwives including Susun Weed, Aviva Romm, Rosemary Gladstar and Gail Faith Edwards.

As always, follow your intuition! Your body has an innate intelligence, and knows what is nourishing and what is not. Use that intelligence when it comes to herbs in the same way that you would use it when it comes to food. Each woman is unique and has a unique relationship to different herbs.

"Just as each person is different and unique, so are herbs. An herbs effect may differ from person to person, but empirical knowledge about herbs is generally true. For centuries, grandmothers have used peppermint tea to ease stomach distress. Chances are good that peppermint will help your stomach feel better too."

~Gail Faith Edwards

Traditional Methods of Preparing Herbal Medicines

Teas & Infusions– Making herbal tea is a really, really enjoyable way of extracting the nourishing and healing properties of herbs. When I was pregnant, I often drank four 16oz jars of different nourishing herbal teas a day. I love preparing and drinking tea – it becomes a ritual and a ceremony that not only nourishes your body, but also your mind and spirit.

When making water-based remedies like teas and infusions, it is usually, (but not always,) best to use dried herbs. For some reason, the process of drying makes nutrients and healing properties release more easily into water. To make a tea or an infusion, boil water in a clean teapot or cooking pot. Place the desired amount of dried herb into a mug or jar which can withstand heat – I always use canning jars. Pour the boiling water into the jar over your herbs. Stir well with a spoon, cover, and let steep.

The difference between a tea and an infusion is the length of time that you steep the herbs. Teas are steeped for a very short time – only 5 to 15 minutes. Some herbs, like chamomile flowers and most seeds, are best steeped as a tea. Most herbs, however, need to be prepared as an infusion. This means that they need to steep at least a few hours in order to extract their nourishing and medicinal properties.

Depending on the type of herb, the number of hours that you let it steep will vary. Flowers need to steep for two hours. Some flowers, like red clover, are best steeped for four hours. Leaves or flowers with leaves attached need to steep at least four hours, and usually longer is better. I often let leaves like nettle and dandelion steep overnight. Roots and barks are the densest parts of the herb, and need to steep the longest in order to extract their medicinal properties. Steep roots and barks for at least eight hours. I will often let these steep overnight or even for a whole day, shaking the jar occasionally once it has cooled completely. (Never shake a jar of hot infusion. The jar will not be able to withstand the pressure of steam released, and it will break and spill hot water everywhere... ummm... Yes... I have done this.)

If you are making a tea/infusion with more than one herb at a time, it is best to use herbs that have compatible steeping times. For example, do not make a tea that contains both fennel seeds and dandelion root. If you steep it for a short amount of time, you won't extract the medicinal properties of the dandelion. If you steep it too long, the fennel seed, which only needs to steep for 20 minutes, will release a bitter taste which doesn't add to its medicinal value. Instead, steep seeds by themselves or with chamomile flowers, with the exception of rose hips which can steep for quite a while. Roots, barks and leaves steep well together.

Once the herbs have steeped, you can strain the infusion through a tea strainer or by hand. I usually squeeze every last drop of water out of the plant material before I compost it.

Infusions can be drunk cold or re-warmed in a pot on the stove. Once herbs have steeped, I like to warm them, add a teaspoon of honey and a dash of raw milk, and relax while I drink. I usually save my tea-drinking times for when my children are asleep and the house is quiet. There is nothing as nourishing for me as this ritual.

Decoctions & Syrups – Decoctions and syrups are also water-based remedies, but are more concentrated and potent than teas and infusions. Decoctions are most often made from dense roots and bark. There are two ways to make a decoction. The first way is add a large handful of your chosen herb to a pot of water. Bring to boil and let simmer on a very low heat for a few hours, until the liquid has reduced by at least half. The second method, which I greatly prefer, is to make a decoction from an infusion. I feel like this method preserves more of the medicinal value in the end result. After infusing an herb and straining out the plant material, add the infusion to a pot. Turn on the heat to the lowest possible setting. Ideally, the infusion should never come to a boil or even a simmer, but should slowly evaporate until it has reduced by half. My favorite herb to make into a decoction is dandelion root – it is nourishing, healing, and with milk and honey I find it to be incredibly delicious.

A syrup is made from a decoction. To make a syrup, add honey, maple syrup or molasses to a warm decoction and stir until it combines with the liquid. Usually you add 4oz to 6oz of honey for each cup of decoction. A syrup will store well in the refrigerator for a few months, and I usually eat a teaspoon or a tablespoon at a time. You can also add syrups to cereal, warm milk, or warm tea.

Tinctures – Tinctures are alcohol-based herbal extracts. You can make tinctures with fresh or dried herbs, but often fresh yields a more potent tincture. Tinctures have many benefits. Although they do not extract much of the nutritive qualities of an herb, they concentrate the medicinal properties and once they are made, they are very easy to use whenever they are needed. Unlike water-based herbal remedies which enter the body more slowly and are better suited for nourishment and healing over time, tinctures are fast acting and can be beneficial in acute situations where a remedy is needed immediately. (For example, in a situation where a hemorrhage seems likely after the birth of the placenta, "shepherd's purse" is often used in the form of a tincture to promote blood clotting and stop the hemorrhage. If shepherd's purse was taken as a tea, the results would be slower-acting and not as effective for that particular situation.) Lastly, once made, tinctures store well for a few years without losing their potency.

Methods vary from plant to plant, but generally speaking, if you're using fresh herbs you chop the plant material coarsely and fill a canning jar with it. Then, pour 100 proof alcohol to the rim of the jar and cap the jar. 100 proof alcohol makes a tincture that is 50% alcohol and 50% water, which is generally desirable. The desired ratio varies slightly from plant to plant. If you use alcohol that is higher proof, you will want to add some pure water to your tincture to obtain a similar water to alcohol ratio. Store the jar in a dark place for six weeks.

If you choose to use dried herbs, you need only fill the jar ¾ of the way to the top, or ½ of the way to the top if you're using dry roots. Follow the same method above, but you'll also want to shake the jar often, even daily, once it's infusing in the alcohol.

Again, the exact method can vary from plant to plant, so if you want to make the perfect tincture than do a little research into the herb that you want to use and the exact ratios of herb to alcohol to water that make the best tinctures.

Oils & Salves – Herbal oils are most often made to be used externally to soothe irritated skin or speed the healing of wounds. To make herbal oil, you can use fresh or dried herbs. When using fresh herbs, always collect the plant on a dry day and let them wilt slightly. Chop the plant coarsely and pack it loosely into a jar. Fill jar most of the way with oil, (olive is best,) and use a spoon to release any air bubbles. Fill the rest of the way – to the rim – with oil and cap the jar. Store in a cool & dark place for four to six weeks. Store the jar on a saucer if you don't want some oil to leak out onto whatever surface it is on. If mold grows in the oil, discard it. After six weeks, strain the herbs. Another way of extracting herbs in oil is through heat. You can use the heat of the sun in a warm windowsill and infuse the herbs in the oil for two weeks before straining, or you can set the jar of herbs/oil in a double boiler or a pot of water in a warm oven and infuse herbs in a few hours to a day. Use your intuition to determine the best method.

Salves are made from herbal oils. I prefer salves to plain herbal oils because they are easier to apply and seem to have better staying power than the oil alone. To make a salve, add 1 part beeswax to a glass jar. Melt the beeswax in the jar by placing the jar in a double boiler. Add 3 parts herbal oil or oils to the jar, and let that warm in the double boiler until you can stir the beeswax and oil together. Once mixed, let cool and use as needed.

Vinegars – Make herbal vinegars when you want to extract the optimum vitamin and mineral content from an herb. Nettle and Dandelion both have a high mineral content and are good herbs to extract in vinegar. Herbal vinegars can be used on salads or cooked greens to add "a boost of flavor and nutrients," as Gail Faith

Edwards says. Raw Apple Cider Vinegar is the best kind vinegar to use. You should only make herbal vinegars from freshly gathered herbs. You can chop the herbs or add them to a jar whole, then cover the herbs with vinegar. Cover the jar with paper or cloth. Do not use metal lids. In place of an herb, you can also extract the minerals from clean egg shells and clean animal bones with vinegar. These vinegars are excellent for remineralizing your own teeth and bones, and improving your overall health.

Honeys – Honey is a very nice way to extract the flavor and medicinal properties of some herbs, and has amazing healing benefits of its own. Use fresh herbs when making herbal honey. Chop them and add them to a jar. Pour fresh raw honey over the herb. When raw honey is fresh, it is still liquid. Once it has crystallized, it is not as easy. You can very gently warm honey that has crystallized in a warm water bath to liquefy it. Be careful not to heat it too much or you will destroy its medicinal properties. Stir the herb into the honey until it is mixed well, and store for at least six weeks before eating. Herbal honeys can last for several years. You can eat herbal honeys plain, add them to teas, or eat them with bread. Some herbs that make good herbal honeys are rose, lemon balm, red clover, garlic, echinacea, bee balm, and ginger, but experiment with other herbs to find out what you enjoy.

A List of Tonic Herbs to Nourish & Support a Healthy Pregnancy

Nettle – Nettle is one of the most nourishing herbs I know of, and my favorite pregnancy tonic! Nettle is incredibly rich in vitamins, minerals, and chlorophyll, and is a supreme tonic for the uterus & hormonal system. It strengthens the kidneys, which are working overtime during pregnancy due to increase in blood volume. With high iron content, nettles can also alleviate nausea & exhaustion associated with anemia. Nettles are also rich in vitamin K, which is important for preventing postpartum hemorrhage as it plays a role in the formation of blood clots. Drink nettle tea regularly to gain the most benefit. Steep the dried leaves for at least four hours to extract all the healing, nourishing qualities, or use the young fresh leaves in cooking – they are delicious. I can't stress enough the amazing nourishment that nettles provide for pregnant (and non-pregnant) women. When I was pregnant, I tried to drink a quart of nettle infusion every day, and found that on days when I met this goal, I had more energy and vitality. It is especially delicious warmed, with a spoonful of honey mixed in and a dash of milk or cream.

Red Raspberry Leaf – Raspberry leaf is widely renowned as a tonic herb for pregnant woman. It is a reproductive & uterine tonic – it strengthens the uterine muscles and prepares the body for childbirth. It is high in calcium, magnesium, and many other minerals & vitamins. It makes a delicious astringent tea, too. I love to use it in combination with other herbs, like nettle, rose, oats, and lemon balm.

Rose – Rose is a beautiful, gentle, & healing herb, and can be used in many ways to support a healthy pregnancy. Rose fruit, (rose hips,) are incredibly rich in vitamin C, and so nourishing & delicious. They can be eaten freshly picked from the bush, dried and steeped in tea, or made into jam. Rose petals have one of the most beautiful smells of any flower, which in and of itself is healing, uplifting, and nourishing to the spirit. Rose petals can be made into a soothing, aromatic & slightly astringent tea, which, apart from nourishing the soul with its beautiful smell and color, also nourishes the body. Rose "hydrosol water" is amazing when used on the skin – it softens and heals dry or irritated skin, which can be helpful during pregnancy. Some types of rose, usually those with ornamental appeal, are less medicinally potent than the simple wild roses, which usually only have five petals on each flower.

Dandelion Leaf & Root – Dandelion is very nourishing, incredibly healing, delicious, and can be used fresh in cooking or dried for tea. Dandelion helps to nourish and support a healthy pregnancy in many ways. It is an incredibly versatile herb, and is quickly becoming one of my closest allies. The roots are supreme liver tonics, and can be of great help during pregnancy since during this time, the liver is working for two! Dandelion supplies abundant potassium, vitamin A, phosphorus, manganese, and iron. It helps to keep the heart healthy, nourishes the blood, kidneys, stomach, and pancreas, and is a lymphatic and immune system tonic. Dandelion is easily recognizable and seems to grow everywhere. It is especially abundant in gardens and fields. When I was growing up, it was one of my favorite flowers! Dandelion can be made into and used as an infusion, decoction, tincture, vinegar, or honey, or can be added to soups and stir fries.

Partridge Berry – Partridge Berry, also known as "Squaw Vine," is an excellent uterine tonic. Herbalists don't seem to agree whether this herb should be used throughout pregnancy or only in the last trimester. It is an excellent late pregnancy tonic when used during the last six weeks of gestation. It can be made into a tea, (steeped for only 15 minutes,) or used as a tincture. Susun Weed writes that "*some midwives use squaw vine only when uterine 'weakness' is indicated by irregular periods, or bleeding during the first trimester. Healthy, full-term, no problem pregnancies are the result.*"

Alfalfa – Alfalfa is considered a good pregnancy tonic herb because of its very high vitamin, mineral, and chlorophyll content. The nourishment it provides strengthens the body and helps to protect against vitamin and mineral deficiencies.

Burdock Root – Burdock root is a supreme liver and blood tonic herb, and can help to support a healthy pregnancy. It is rich in minerals, too, and is a mild digestive stimulant and laxative. Burdock is best used as an infusion or decoction, but can also be used as a tincture. The roots are delicious in stir-fries.

Oats – Oats, which include all aerial parts of the plant including the grain we eat as cereal, support a well-nourished mother in many ways. For one, they are an excellent nervine tonic. Think of how you feel after eating a bowl of warm oatmeal – relaxed, calm, and maybe even a little sleepy. This relaxation is often much needed during pregnancy. Oats also supply calcium and magnesium. Besides oatmeal, oats or oat-straw can also be made into an infusion or a tincture that can be used daily.

Yellow Dock – Yellow dock is high in iron and an excellent liver tonic. Yellow dock root has helped me through a few rough situations in my pregnancies, and I am so grateful. I've used it to assist in easing exhaustion, anemia, & nausea, with really, really amazing results. Apart from its high iron content, yellow dock is also high in many other minerals, supports hormonal balance, and is a mild laxative.

Wild, Home-Grown, or Purchased?

Where do you go when you are in search of an herb?

Wild-Gathering herbs always yields the most potent, vital, and healing herbs. Herbs that grow in the wild are allowed to put down their roots where they choose, and the result is a plant that, as Matthew Wood says, *"lives in and adapts to the environmental stresses and niches"* that they are designed for. These environmental factors result in an incredibly potent life-energy in the plant. *"The triumphs of their life force over the adversities of nature are etched into their genetic makeup"* and this amplifies the quality of their medicinal properties. Anyone who has tasted the difference between the little vital dandelion leaves, plucked fresh from a wild meadow or streamside, and the sort of enormous bland dandelion leaves that you can purchase at Whole Foods that come from shipped from California, knows the difference that I am speaking of. Those little wild dandelions have so much life-energy, and are so incredibly potent when compared with the dandelions that are cultivated commercially and shipped long distances before arriving at market.

Wild gathering, apart from bearing potent herbs, also has the benefit of letting you get to know the plants. The medicine that plants have to offer is not just in their chemical constituents, or their vitamins and minerals. Plants also offer advice and remedy through their living presence. Connecting to the plants that you choose to use as remedies can be a great gift.

When you wild-gather, make sure you can easily identify the plant you are looking for. Some plants, like Stinging Nettles and Dandelions, are extremely easy to identify and abundant in many parts of the world. Others are more subtle, and some have look-alikes that can be potentially harmful or, dare I say, fatal, so learn to identify plants correctly before making them into medicine. Always harvest wild herbs from uncontaminated wild locations. Herbs growing by roads and train tracks are not suited for medicine, at least internal medicine. These plants still offer their spiritual remedies, though.

"Learning to recognize herbs in the wild is far easier, and much less fraught with danger, than most people realize… Even if you never pick your own herbs, knowing how the live plants look will be a great asset when you go out to buy them."

~ Susun Weed

Cultivating herbs in a garden or in pots at home is a beautiful way to get to know herbs, and this method often yields very potent herbs as well. Although these herbs may not have the same powerful & vital spark as the herbs that grow wild, they will have a very intimate relationship with you as their cultivator, and this is not something to be overlooked when it comes to their medicinal and nutritive value.

Plants change in response to their environment. No two dandelions are the same. Plants that you cultivate will change specifically in their relationship with you. Many traditional cultures speak of the necessity of talking to the plants – of asking plants to fill the empty spaces in your body or heal the imbalanced aspects of yourself before harvesting and making these plants into medicine. For many of us modern humans this may sound like superstition. However, even science now shows that plants can and do alter their chemical makeup in response to their environment, including human interactions. A plant that you have grown yourself and developed an intimate relationship with will know better how to heal and nourish you!

Buying herbs is a good option, too. There are many small family herb growers & gatherers who are so glad to share their herbs, and their knowledge. It's nice to buy from the smaller "family" growers/gatherers, because this supports their passion and supports a future with plentiful local herbalists and herb-gatherers. If you can't find an herb or a tincture through a small or local herbal business, big herb companies like Mountain Rose sell massive quantities of herbs and have huge selections – chances are they have what you're looking for. When you buy herbs, make sure that they are as fresh as possible as well as wild-harvested or organically cultivated.

Herbal & Nutritional Remedies for Common Pregnancy Problems

Women often experience nausea, exhaustion, indigestion, and a variety of ailments during pregnancy. The best way to avoid the common ailments of pregnancy is through a healthy diet, fresh air, sunlight, friendship, love, joy, plenty of sleep, and adequate movement. Some of these ailments, morning sickness for example, are so common that they have come to be considered a normal part of pregnancy.

In traditional cultures, these ailments were seemingly unheard of. Our world today is very different from the world of our ancestors and some might say it is a less hospitable world for a pregnant woman. Still, excellent self-care through all kinds of nourishment, including nutritious foods and *tonic* herbs, is the best way to prevent these ailments.

When an ailment does occur, it is often a sign that something is out of balance. Imbalances can occur on many levels – they can be physical, emotional, mental, or spiritual. An ailment is a symptom of the imbalance, rather than the imbalance itself. Addressing only the physical symptoms will only ever provide temporary relief. (Sometimes temporary relief can be an amazing and beautiful thing.) When these ailments occur, however, it is a beautiful opportunity to learn about yourself. It grants you the chance to look within to find the true cause of the imbalance, and it presents you with the opportunity to heal yourself on a deeper level. Once you have found the root of the imbalance and addressed it, lasting relief from the symptoms is much easier to obtain.

Herbal medicine has the potential to both help provide temporary relief of symptoms and to address those deeper imbalances. I strongly caution, however, against using herbs only to address the symptoms without taking a deeper look at the underlying causes of the symptoms. Herbs are great allies to those who practice a lifestyle of self-care. They never replace self-care.

Susun Weed, who advocates for a very gentle approach to wellness and health care, has an excellent system for addressing an issue when it arises. She calls this system the "six steps of healing." There are actually seven steps, because the first step, "step 0," involves "doing nothing." Doing nothing does not mean that you continue life as usual, for this is potentially what caused the issue in the first place. "Do nothing" means rest, relax, turn off the computer and unplug the phone. Turn off the lights and turn off your mind. Simply be, and *do* nothing. It is not until the fourth step, "step 3," that Susun Weed suggests introducing the use of physical herbal medicine. You can find more on this method with a quick google search, or through Susun Weed's books.

My reason for sharing Susun's method is this: it demonstrates that we all too often jump to using medicines, herbal or otherwise, to treat our symptoms or our ailments without first taking a good critical look at our lifestyle, feelings, and thoughts. Herbal medicines can help us tremendously with so many things, but not if we use them to replace healthy self-care. Keep this in mind when you are reading through the following list of herbs and herbal remedies for some of the common ailments of pregnancy:

Table of Contents forHerbal & Nutritional Remedies for Common Pregnancy Problems:

Anemia

Anemia refers to the symptoms experienced when a person is deficient in red blood cells. Usually anemia is caused by a deficiency of Iron, Folic Acid, or Vitamin B12. Anemic people can exhibit mild to extreme fatigue, paleness, dizziness, poor appetite and digestion, trouble breathing and heart palpitations.

Anemia should be easy to remedy through dietary changes and herbal remedies. Depending on the type of anemia, the protocol is different. For Iron Deficiency Anemia, make sure to include iron-rich foods and herbs in your diet. These include kale, red meats, dried fruits like figs and prunes, molasses, kidney beans, nettle leaves, dandelion, yellow dock, and eggs. Make sure to support your liver, which regulates iron levels in the body. Herbs that support the liver include yellow dock root, dandelion root, and burdock root. Include foods that contain vitamin C in your diet, and eat vitamin C-rich foods along with Iron-rich foods, because vitamin C helps the body absorb iron.

I realized that iron-deficiency anemia was the cause of my exhaustion about a month or two into my second pregnancy. I was completely unable to function. All I wanted to do was sleep, but that was hard to do with my one-year-old daughter to care for. Once I realized I was anemic, I prepared the "iron tonic syrup" that Aviva Romm and many other herbalists suggest for iron deficiency. (It is so easy to make: Prepare a decoction of yellow dock root, and then make a syrup using molasses. Instructions on making a decoction & Syrup are in the previous chapter.) The iron tonic syrup eaten daily, coupled with daily nettle tea and some minor dietary changes, helped tremendously, and within a week or two I was feeling my energy levels return to normal!

Vitamin B12 Deficiency can also cause anemia, and can be remedied trough adding B12 rich foods to the diet. Animal foods and bacteria are shown to be the only bioavailable source of vitamin B12. Good quality meats have much greater amounts of B12 than poor quality meats. B12 can be stored in the body for up to 5 years, but after 5 years without the nutrient, B12 deficiency can appear. Stored B12 may not reach the developing fetus in the same way that regularly consumed B12 would do.

Deficiency in Folic Acid, another B vitamin, can also cause anemia. Remedies are herbs and foods high in folic acid. These include leafy greens like kale, root vegetables, grass-fed milk, liver, nutritional yeast, molasses, amaranth, nettles, dandelion and lamb's quarters.

Exhaustion & Fatigue

Fatigue is an issue that many women face in pregnancy. It can be brought on by many factors – anemia, lack of adequate sleep, poor nutrition, stress, lack of fresh air or exercise, being over-worked, depression, or lack of motivation & drive. Because of the wide range of causes, there are many ways to remedy fatigue.

Herbal stimulants are not recommended during pregnancy. Stimulants provide temporary energy, but often if fatigue is present during pregnancy what is really needed is not an energy boost, but a slow and nourishing regimen of self-care.

If fatigue is persistent, debilitating, and is accompanied by symptoms of anemia, see the section on the three common types of anemia, listed above. If fatigue is due to lack of sleep, then the only true remedy is to find ways to get more sleep. Take naps if possible. Go to bed an hour earlier every evening. If you experience insomnia or stress that is causing fatigue, then see the section on "insomnia & anxiety" in the following pages.

If fatigue is due to an excessive workload, then do what you can to reduce the workload. Ask for help from friends or relatives to ease your load. Pregnant women need a good support network.

If lack of fresh air and exercise are the problem, then make time to immerse yourself in nature and go for walks. Walking in nature can greatly alleviate depression and restore a sense of purpose and motivation as well.

If fatigue is due to inadequate nutrition, then take a look at your diet. Often eating a protein-rich snack will help immensely in alleviating fatigue. Make sure you are eating enough, and not skipping meals due to stress or a heavy workload. I noticed in my second pregnancy that if I ate melon for my mid-morning snack, I would become incredibly fatigued and even nauseous shortly thereafter. The melon just didn't meet my nutritional requirements at that time. When I replaced the melon with a big bowl of yogurt with walnuts and blueberries and granola, my energy levels never took that dive.

Many tonic herbs, which nourish your whole pregnant body, will help to provide you with overall energy and vitality when used over time. Make it a practice to drink at least one, if not multiple cups of nettle, dandelion, raspberry or alfalfa infusion each day.

Digestive Complaints

Digestive complaints can include heartburn, constipation, gas and bloating, or diarrhea. A loving and stress-free relationship to your food is the number one remedy for digestive complaints. Chew slowly – enjoy mealtimes – don't hurry or worry as you eat. Eat when you are hungry and choose foods that you really, really love or desire.

Heartburn seems to occur for many women in late pregnancy. It can be caused by anxiety, excess or too little stomach acid, or the displacement and constriction of the stomach due to your growing belly. Heartburn can be alleviated by eating small meals slowly, with shorter intervals between the meals, rather than a few large meals eaten all at once. You can also make digestive teas from carminative seeds like anise, fennel, or dill. Add a teaspoon of honey and a dash of milk, which can also help alleviate heartburn. Sip the tea slowly before, during, and especially after meals. A deficiency in natural salt may also contribute to heartburn.

Susun Weed suggests using a teaspoon of slippery elm bark powder, mixed with honey, just after meals to alleviate heartburn. slippery elm soothes the stomach and the intestines, and is often used as a food and remedy for people who experience severe digestive problems. Slippery Elm can also alleviate gas and bloating.

Constipation is common in pregnancy, and can sometimes cause pain or discomfort. First, ask yourself: What are you afraid to let go of? Are you holding on to something? Second, gentle movement, exercise, and adequate water intake can all help alleviate constipation. Thirdly, too little food can contribute to constipation, so make sure that you are eating enough. And finally, there are gentle and safe dietary and herbal remedies which can alleviate the discomfort and keep your digestion moving regularly.

Homemade soups, cooked figs, raisins, and prunes, oatmeal, and fresh salad greens can all be added to your diet if you wish to improve the flow of your digestion. Herbs like yellow dock root and dandelion root, prepared as a decoction or a syrup with molasses, are excellent for stimulating digestive movement. They can be used regularly during pregnancy – one or two tablespoons of syrup or a half-cup of decoction each day. Never use commercial or harsh herbal laxatives like senna or cascara sagrada during pregnancy.

Diarrhea, although not as common as constipation, can also occur in pregnancy. Chronic diarrhea can cause nutrient loss and dehydration, and can be a real problem for mother and baby. If you experience chronic diarrhea during pregnancy, take a really good look at your diet to see if there are any hard-to-digest foods which might be the cause. (I experienced chronic diarrhea after the birth of my first daughter, and until I completely eliminated nuts and all whole grains from my diet, it did not stop. It was debilitating and exhausting. A bit later, I was able to re-introduce some nuts and grains. Now, as long as I don't eat un-sprouted whole grains, I never have a problem.)

If you experience bouts of mild diarrhea, there are tonifying and astringent herbs that can be very helpful. Red raspberry leaf, blackberry leaf or rose petals are all astringent herbs and help to tone the intestinal lining, which in turn improves digestion and normal bowel movements. Make a strong infusion of any of these herbs and use until diarrhea subsides. If these herbs don't help, the best herb to tonify the intestines and relieve diarrhea is blackberry root. Make a decoction and drink ¼ cup at a time, with a little honey, until diarrhea subsides.

Backaches & Muscle Cramps

Although these ailments have many causes, there are some general herbal and dietary recommendations that can help to alleviate them. If backache is caused by kidney stress, you can make some dietary changes and use nourishing herbs to support kidney health. First, try not to drink cold liquids like ice water or cold juice, which can be hard on the kidneys. Instead, eat & drink warming and nourishing foods and beverages. Nettle leaf is a perfect pregnancy herb for nourishing the kidneys and helping them to function optimally. Drink nettle infusion warmed with a bit of honey. Also, any pregnancy herb which supplies calcium & magnesium, like oat-straw, can be very helpful. Susun Weed also suggests comfrey infusion, which she says "provides every vitamin and mineral necessary to prevent backaches."

If backache is caused by a bladder infection, see the section on "Urinary Tract and Bladder Infections" in the coming pages.

Gentle exercise and regular movement can be helpful for alleviating cramps and aches. Making love with your partner or going for a walk everyday are both great ways to accomplish this. However, if aches and cramps are caused by too much strenuous movement, than rest is necessary.

Ask your partner or your friends to give you back and leg massages, which can release tension, relieve pain and be extremely relaxing and nourishing for pregnant mothers. Also, make sure your intestines are working well and that you are not constipated. If constipation is causing backache, see the section on "Digestive Complaints" above.

Some herbal remedies can be very helpful in relieving pain safely. Tincture of cramp bark, as its name implies, can be used to relieve muscle cramps and back spasms. According to Aviva Romm, you can take up to 25 drops of cramp bark tincture every half-hour for no more than 2 hours. Alternatively, you can use 25 drops up to 4 times a day.

You can also use herbs externally to relieve pain – st. john's wort-infused oil, massaged into painful areas, alone or as a salve, can help reduce pain as well as inflammation. You can take herbal baths with gentle and relaxing herbs like rose, chamomile, oats, and lemon balm. You can either make a strong infusion of the dried herbs and add it to your bath, or put the dry herbs into a little mesh bag, tie it to the faucet of your bath, and let the hot water stream through it as the bath fills. Not only do the smells of the herbs rise with the steam and create a beautifully relaxing atmosphere, but once you're in the bath, you absorb the relaxing and soothing properties of the herbs through your skin. You can also add Epsom or Dead Sea salts to your bath, and a splash of apple cider vinegar. Bath salts help to relax muscles, promote deep relaxation, and detoxify the body, and they are safe to use while pregnant. To use, dissolve a cup of salt in a warm (not hot) bath. Bathe for not more than 20 minutes, and then rinse off briefly in the shower. If you want to take a longer bath, just add the salts near the end of the bath, 15 minutes before you want to get out. Be careful, however, to only use plain bath salt – do not use bath salts that have added essential oils or other components that could potentially be harmful during pregnancy.

Gentle nervine tonics drunk as infusions, like oats, skullcap, and lemon balm, can also help to relax the body and support the relief of back pain and muscle cramps. These can also be used as tinctures. (If you have low thyroid function then avoid skullcap and lemon balm.)

Morning sickness

Morning sickness is often considered the most common complication of early pregnancy. It can be debilitating and exhausting, and doesn't necessarily happen only in the morning. For some women it can last all day. If vomiting accompanies the nausea, which is the case for some women, it can deplete your body of nutrients as well.

Low blood sugar is a very common cause of morning sickness, but not the only cause. Morning sickness can be caused by hormonal imbalances, vitamin and mineral deficiencies, poor eating habits, normal changes in the digestive system, and lack of self-care. Your emotional response to being pregnant also plays a role – if your pregnancy something that is hard to digest, so to say, than this emotional reaction may be manifesting as nausea.

Morning sickness can be prevented, diminished, or alleviated by eating nutritious and appetizing protein-rich meals often throughout the day, drinking herbal tonic infusions regularly, getting lots of fresh air and sunlight, being active, sleeping well, and drinking digestive teas and infusions.

By eating nutritious meals often, you ensure that your body has lasting energy and enough vitamins, minerals, and protein to continue to grow your baby! Eating fruit by itself, or eating other snacks that contain only simple sugars, is not the best choice for all pregnant women. They will give you a short spurt of energy that will quickly drop, leaving you hungry before you even know it. This is often a cause of fatigue, nausea, and even vomiting. Add yogurt or cottage cheese or another substantial food to snacks that are made up of only simple sugars to help prevent morning sickness.

By drinking herbal tonic infusions regularly, you ensure that you are getting an abundant supply of vitamins and minerals. Deficiencies in iron, calcium, magnesium, B vitamins, and many other nutrients can cause morning sickness, which is why nausea often accompanies anemia. Nettle leaves, red raspberry leaves, and dandelion leaves and roots are my favorite herbs to use to supply abundant nutrients to ease morning sickness. Drink multiple cups of infusion every day for the best results. Yellow dock root is another herb that supplies abundant nutrients, especially iron. A combination of yellow dock root syrup and nettle leaf infusion, coupled with lots of sunlight and fresh air over the course of a week, helped my morning sickness disappear.

If you are nauseous and looking for immediate relief, there are some digestive herbs that can liberate you from that awful discomfort. The first, and my favorite, is ginger. You can make an infusion of fresh or dried ginger root and drink slowly, sipping to alleviate nausea. Ginger root in combination with dandelion root also works very well. This infusion works best when it is warmed and a teaspoon of honey added. However, ginger is a uterine stimulant, and therefore should be used with caution, particularly in the first trimester or by women who have miscarried. Carminative seeds like anise, fennel, and dill can be helpful too. Steep a tablespoon of these seeds for 15 minutes, add a bit of honey, and drink slowly. Mints like peppermint or spearmint are also effective at relieving nausea.

Miscarriage

Miscarriage is something that I do not have personal experience with, at least as far as I am aware. I have read many personal stories of miscarriage and loss in the first 20 weeks of pregnancy, but I do not claim to know the experience. I felt, however, that leaving the topic of miscarriage out of this book would be doing a disservice to you as the reader. I have decided to include information on miscarriage based on my readings in Aviva Romm's "Natural Pregnancy Book" and Susun Weed's "Herbal for the Childbearing Year." Aviva devotes 14 pages in her book to the prevention of a threatened miscarriage, what to do if a miscarriage can't be prevented, and what to do after a miscarriage. Her description is very thorough and written from her experience as a midwife, and for anyone who wishes to know more than I provide here, I would suggest her book.

Miscarriage Prevention: Signs of a possible miscarriage include bleeding and lower back cramps in early pregnancy. Aviva Romm stresses the value of communicating with your baby during this time. "Your desire to continue the pregnancy will support your efforts.... you can communicate your desire to have the baby, also giving the baby permission to go if he or she needs to." She and Susun Weed agree that bed rest is extremely important. Aviva also suggests warm baths and stresses the importance of only eating warm foods and consuming warm drinks. "It takes a certain degree of warmth in the womb, not unlike incubating eggs until they hatch."

Both Susun and Aviva suggest that black haw root bark infusion is an excellent miscarriage preventative. It can be used daily, beginning as soon as you are pregnant and can be used throughout the entire pregnancy. Susun suggests "one or two cups of tea or a half cup of the infusion daily." Susun also suggests that if you have experienced repeated miscarriages, false unicorn root may help "even when the cervix is too loose to hold the pregnancy." Her suggested dose is "3 drops of tincture, 4 to 5 times daily, beginning a month before conception and continuing for the entire first trimester." Susun cautions, however, that false unicorn is a very powerful herb and should not be used without the guidance of an experienced herbalist.

Partridge berry (or squaw vine,) wild yam root, lobelia, and vitex berry (or chasteberry) are all herbs that can be used safely to help prevent miscarriage as well. Aviva Romm suggests that for women with a history of miscarriage, a tincture mixture can be made using "1 ounce cramp bark or black haw, 1 ounce chasteberry, 1 ounce wild yam, ½ ounce partridge berry, ¼ ounce lobelia, and ¼ ounce ginger." She suggests mixing all of these tinctures together and taking "1/2 to 1 teaspoon twice daily for preventative care," and if a miscarriage begins, increasing the dose to "1/2 to 1 teaspoon every 15 minutes to every 2 hours" depending on the "severity and frequency of the contractions." Aviva suggests that you continue to use this mixture (at the 'preventative' dosage) until two weeks after the point at which you miscarried in your previous pregnancy. Susun Weed also suggests that a sip of whisky or another alcohol will stop contractions.

If a miscarriage cannot be prevented: Both Susun Weed and Aviva Romm emphasize the importance of having someone by your side if you are experiencing a miscarriage. Since your body has not yet built up to the 50% blood increase that is present after mid-term, miscarriage carries a greater risk of hemorrhage and shock. Aviva says that "A normal miscarriage tends to have more continuous bleeding than a normal birth….Your vitality and coherence as well as how long and how much you've been bleeding are good indications of how you are doing."

Aviva advises seeking professional help if you are bleeding heavily for more than 2 hours without successfully miscarrying, but that you will probably be ok to continue the miscarriage without professional help if bleeding is mild, even if your cramps are strong. Aviva describes heavy bleeding as "soaking a medium-sized sanitary pad in thirty minutes."

For a miscarriage to end, the uterus needs to empty completely. Until then, cramping and bleeding will continue.

Susun Weed's herbal advice for completing a miscarriage is to "have herbs which control bleeding on hand" and "use 20 drops each of blue and black cohosh tinctures every hour to empty the uterus. Do not exceed five doses. To control bleeding, use 10-20 drops of shepherd's purse tincture… under the tongue as often as needed."

Aviva also suggests not sleeping while you are bleeding, keeping warm and continuing to drink liquids often, peeing when you need to, visualizing your womb successfully emptying, and listening to the cues of your body. Essentially, miscarriage is similar in many ways to giving birth – your body goes through the same motions in miscarriage as it would birthing a full-term baby.

Post-Miscarriage: "Essentially," as Aviva says, "you have gone through birth without getting a baby." This makes bodily, hormonal, and emotional adjustment to your non-pregnant state quite difficult.

After a miscarriage, "your immediate concerns are infection and bleeding."Aviva suggests using "15 to 20 drops 3 times daily" of angelica tincture to ensure that the uterus is fully cleared, and using "1 teaspoon of echinacea four times daily to stimulate your immune response and as a preventative against infection." She says that 10 drops of calendula tincture can be used with every teaspoon of echinacea, along with "2,000 mg of vitamin C over the course of each day." Change your menstrual pad very often – every few hours – and refrain from sex until bleeding has completely stopped. Nourish yourself during this period, in all ways.

Varicose Veins & Hemorrhoids

Varicosities during pregnancy are somewhat common, especially for women whose mothers and grandmothers also experienced them. I had no problem with them during my first two pregnancies, but experienced vulvar varicosities in my third pregnancy. I felt a lot of pressure in my vagina, but I didn't even know I had varicosities until I examined with a hand mirror. It made sex uncomfortable and I needed to rest more often so as not to aggravate them. It also felt embarrassing, and for a while I didn't even want to talk about it with friends.

Varicosities are caused by poor circulation or weakness in the blood's capacity to flow easily through the veins. Blood builds up in certain areas, further weakening and distending the veins, and does not easily return to the heart - this causes varicose veins. For pregnant women, this occurs especially in the lower parts of the body: the legs, groin, vulva and anus. When varicosities appear in the anus, they are called hemorrhoids. Sometimes, varicosities do not appear until just after giving birth.

Varicosities can be made worse by long periods of standing, especially standing still. A simple and obvious way to help prevent varicose veins is to invert your body so that the lower parts are above your heart, rather than below. This gives the blood in the lower parts a chance to flow more easily back to the heart, and prevents blood from pooling in the lower body. You don't have to stand on your head to do this, although that can apparently help; try lying on your back and propping your butt and legs up as high as you can, with your knees bent comfortably, and rest for a few minutes to let your circulation balance itself. It helps, at least to provide temporary relief. Be creative and find other ways to do this that feel good to your body & relieve the pressure in your lower parts.

Stay active; a sedentary lifestyle can worsen varicose veins. Walking, bike-riding, swimming and hiking can help – anything that gets your heart thumping just a little more powerfully. Diet can also assist: Susun weed suggests garlic & onions, oats, leafy green vegetables, beets, and any foods rich in vitamins A, E, and C, as well as B vitamins to help the circulatory and elimination systems. She suggests avoiding cayenne, black pepper, curries and hot spices, since these "increase congestion in the offending veins, often causing bleeding in hemorrhoids." A specific bioflavonoid called Rutin is also said to be greatly effective.

Any herbs that aid the heart, circulatory system, or the digestive system are helpful for varicose veins. Herbs (and doses) to use to support these systems include 30 drops every the morning and evening of hawthorn and dandelion root tinctures, multiple cups a day of nettle leaf infusion (you can add oatstraw to the infusion too,) and even a few drops, two or three times a day, of motherwort tincture as long as you use it sparingly and do not use it until after the first trimester, (Motherwort is considered by some to be an emmenagogue.) Be wary of combining motherwort and hawthorn, as this can lower blood pressure so much as to cause dizziness.

For external relief of varicose veins, try applying a witch hazel or white oak bark compress in problematic areas. The astringency of witch hazel & white oak help in two ways: they relieve pain & swelling, and they tighten and tone the veins and tissues surrounding the veins. Aviva Romm suggests that wrapping the affected areas with a cloth soaked in an astringent extract is safer than massaging the area. Make a strong infusion of these herbs, or as Aviva suggests, simmer them for 30 minutes in a covered pot, let cool until they reach a tolerable temperature, and then apply to your varicosities for 20 minute intervals by wrapping with a cloth. I soaked a cloth menstrual pad in which hazel extract and applied it each night for 15 minutes, which I found to provide great relief.

If your varicose veins don't disappear, don't stress. Sometimes they stick around until after the baby is born no matter what you do.

Colds & Mild Illness during Pregnancy

You can help to prevent colds and mild illnesses during pregnancy by following an overall healthy lifestyle, eating nourishing foods, drinking regular infusions of nettle, dandelion, raspberry and other nourishing tonic herbs, spending time in nature, laughing often, and loving yourself.

If you do get sick, rest, nurture yourself, and stay warm. Staying warm includes eating warming, nourishing foods like soups, stews, and casseroles, and avoiding cold foods. Cold milk, for example, can aggravate illness, while milk that has been gently warmed can be healing. There are also gentle warming herbs that can stimulate movement & healing. Ginger is my favorite, though again, it should be used with caution, especially during the first trimester.

Herbs which support the immune system, like echinacea, as well as nutritive herbs like nettle and dandelion, can all support healing from colds. Echinacea can be taken effectively as a tincture, but a warmed infusion of echinacea root with a teaspoon of honey is better. Honey is also warming and has immune system strengthening properties.

Steams, showers and warm baths can also be immensely helpful at clearing congestion and restoring health.

Urinary Tract Infections & Bladder Infections

Bladder and urinary tract infections (UTI's) occur more often during pregnancy due to extra stress on the kidneys and elimination systems. It is best to treat a UTI as soon as you notice it, otherwise it can worsen and turn into a kidney infection. Symptoms of UTIs include frequent urination (this in and of itself does not mean you have an infection – frequent urination is normal in pregnancy,) lower back or lower abdominal pain, painful urination, and feeling sick.

If you develop a UTI, use immune-supporting herbs like garlic and echinacea. Garlic can be added to cooking and eaten raw if you can stand it. One good way to stomach raw garlic is to float finely minced garlic in water and drink it quickly. To use Echinacea, Aviva Romm suggests "1 drop per 2 pounds of body weight every four hours until symptoms are gone, then 20 drops three times a day for a few more days." Alternative to the tincture, a strong echinacea root infusion can be used. Also, greatly increase your dietary vitamin C intake or use a vitamin C supplement, 1500 to 2000 mg spread throughout the day.

Susun Weed and Aviva Romm both strongly recommend uva ursi, but they both caution not to use it in the first trimester, and to use it with caution thereafter. Susun suggests to "brew 1 ounce of uva ursi leaves in a quart of boiling water for eight hours. Drink one cup of this infusion every 12 hours for the first two days, or, in severe cases, one cup every 4 hours. Continue with at least one cup daily for another three days, even if the symptoms disappear sooner. Do not use uva ursi for more than 10 days." Yarrow can also be used, for no more than five days, in conjunction with uva ursi.

Also, reduce your sugar consumption while you are healing from your UTI, and very importantly, pee when you need to! Holding in your pee is a huge factor in the development of UTIs, and continuing to hold in your pee if you develop a UTI will worsen the infection and oppose the healing process.

Irritability, Anxiety & Insomnia

Excellent self-care and holistic nourishment can have a profound beneficial effect on mood, sleep, and psychological health. Issues with anxiety, irritability and insomnia are often a sign that there is something below the surface that needs expression or acknowledgement – do not neglect this, rather take this time to nourish yourself and to really be honest with yourself about what you and your baby need.

Raspberry and nettle infusions, when consumed regularly, supply abundant minerals which can help immensely. Herbs with plentiful magnesium are also especially helpful for stress and tension release. When magnesium is deficient, the body tends to hold tension more easily, and this can easily manifest as irritability, stress, anxiety and insomnia.

Gentle nervine tonic herbs like skullcap, lemon balm, and oats can be relaxing and helpful for these issues, especially insomnia. Motherwort, one of my favorite herbs, is very helpful for irritability and stress – it doesn't cause tiredness but it supports relaxation, stress release, and tension release. Motherwort should not be used in the first trimester, and it can cause dependency if used too often, so keep that in mind and remember to focus on nourishing yourself emotionally, spiritually, and otherwise before relying on motherwort. You can use about five drops of motherwort tincture at a time, and repeat every two hours, if needed, during times of stress or anxiety.

A good, warm bath is often one of the best remedies for tension release. Add relaxing herbal tea or a bag of bath herbs to the your bath before entering, or a add cup of Epsom or Dead Sea salt near the end of the bath (in the last 20 minutes, and rinse off afterward) for an even more deeply relaxing experience.

Itchiness & Skin Irritation

Itchiness is somewhat common in pregnancy. Your body is going through dramatic changes during this time – it is not uncommon to gain 20, 30, 40, even 50 pounds during pregnancy. Your skin stretches in ways that it never has before, and this can sometimes cause itchiness. If this is the case, herbal infused oils can be of great assistance. Try rose petal or calendula flower-infused oil, made into a cream or "body butter." You can use olive oil to infuse the flowers/petals, and then once it has infused, mix it with shea butter and a bit of beeswax, by using a double boiler. Never heat shea Butter above 150 degrees, since this destroys its healing properties. When the herbal oil has been mixed with the butter or wax, add a few drops of sweet orange essential oil. This body butter will ease dryness and itchiness and deeply nourish skin.

Itchiness can also be a sign of a stressed liver. The liver processes toxins and helps to eliminate them from the body. During pregnancy the liver can become overloaded due to extra hormones and an increased food intake. Toxins instead find a way out through the skin, causing itchiness. If a stressed liver is the problem, then no amount of topically applied oils will really soothe your skin, although they can help in the short term. Herbs and foods that support the liver in functioning optimally are needed here. It is so important to support your liver during pregnancy!

Dandelion root, yellow dock root, and burdock root are all wonderful liver-supporting herbs. Dandelion root tastes wonderful when made into a strong decoction with a bit of honey and milk added. Burdock root has never been one of my favorites because of its strong taste, but I used it copiously as an infusion during pregnancy when I experienced excessive itchiness due to a very overworked liver, and it was a great help. You can make an infusion of any of these three herbs using 1 ounce of root in 1 quart of boiling water, and steeping for at least 8 hours before straining. (Yellow dock tastes much better if it is made into a decoction and then into a syrup using blackstrap molasses.) Milk thistle seed can also be used, either in tincture form or in the form of freshly groundseeds. A coffee grinder works well for grinding whole milk thistle seed. Very rarely, people can be allergic to milk thistle, so if you have a strong reaction then discontinue use.

Short, warm baths with Epsom salt or Dead Sea salt can also be very helpful for drawing out toxins and soothing the skin. Add a cup of salt to a warm bath, and soak no more than 20 minutes before rinsing off. Be aware that Epsom salt baths can lower blood sugar, so have a sweet snack on hand just in case.

High Blood Pressure

The most common causes of high blood pressure are stress, malnutrition, and a sedentary lifestyle. Therefore, lifestyle changes such as taking time to relax, nourishing your emotions, eating a nutritious diet, walking more, swimming, and getting lots of fresh air and sunlight can greatly improve or eliminate high blood pressure, (also called hypertension.) Making this lifestyle a practice throughout pregnancy is a preventative against hypertension.

Adding sea salt to meals, to taste, is also very important in preventing high blood pressure. Conventional medicine often advocates for restricted salt intake, claiming that too much salt will actually cause high blood pressure. This may be true for some people, but only when they eat table salt. Table salt seems to be the standard salt in most American diets. Table salt usually contains very toxic synthetic additives and anti-caking agents. When you eat table salt, it may cause a rise in blood pressure for some people, along with an array of other longer-term health problems. So by all means, do not eat table salt! Sea salt, however, has actually been shown to lower high blood pressure, making it an effective remedy to those with hypertension. Restricting your salt intake during pregnancy is definitely not a good idea, especially if you are worried about hypertension. It is important, however, to ensure that your salt is unprocessed and free of toxic additives.

Getting plenty of fluids throughout the day is important for reducing hypertension. Whether it's through soups, broths, herbal teas or infusions, juice, or just plain water, make sure that you drink plenty. Some sources say ½ gallon a day is recommended in pregnancy. I found this easy, as I would usually drink two quarts of herbal tea throughout the day. However, too much liquid can be as problematic as too little, so listen to your body's needs.

Relaxing herbs can reduce hypertension by reducing stress; chamomile, oats, skullcap, and lemon balm are all relaxing. Motherwort has the benefit of being both relaxing and a beneficial herb for the heart. You can use 5 drops of motherwort tincture a few times a day to help reduce blood pressure, but do not use motherwort in the first trimester, and be aware that some say motherwort can cause dependency. Hawthorn is also a beneficial herb for the heart, and is helpful in reducing hypertension. 30 drops of hawthorn tincture can be taken 2 or 3 times a day.

Minor Swelling

Minor swelling is completely normal during pregnancy. (If swelling is severe, see the section below on "problematic swelling & toxemia.) Feet and ankles are the most commonly affected part of the body during pregnancy.

Taking herbal baths or baths with Epsom or Dead Sea salts can assist greatly if there is discomfort associated with minor swelling. Make sure any bath salts are just plain salt, without essential oils or other ingredients. You can add your own essential oils, but make sure they are safe for use in pregnancy and be aware that most essential oils are extremely concentrated and should be used with care.

Do not restrict your salt intake, as this can greatly aggravate edema and swelling. Make sure, however, that you are eating real high quality sea salt and not table salt. Also, make sure you are eating protein, and plenty of it. Aviva Romm cautions that "inadequate intake of protein and salt is linked with toxemia."

Minor swelling can also be helped by herbs which promote healthy circulation, such as dandelion root and hawthorn, and by herbs which promote proper kidney function, like nettle leaf and dandelion. Dandelion and nettle can be made into infusions or decoctions, 2 cups a day, and hawthorn can be used as a tea, infusion, or a tincture. In Susun Weed's article "Take Heart from Hawthorn," she suggests that *"a dose is a cup of tea, half a cup of infusion, or a dropperful of tincture, taken first thing in the morning and last thing at night. For the first three months of use, a third dose, mid-day, may be added. Traditional European herbalists always add a big spoon of honey to hawthorn tea or infusion."*

Gestational Diabetes (GD)

GD is a commonly diagnosed disease of pregnancy. Many do not question this definition, since blood glucose tests often indicate a rise in blood sugar during pregnancy. What is left out of this, however, is that a normal, healthy pregnancy, by its very nature, involves a steady rise in blood sugar throughout gestation. This rise in blood sugar serves an important purpose – it is especially important for the developing brain of the fetus.

Management of GD based on restricting foods with a high glycemic index has proved ineffectual time and time again, and management of GD based in insulin supplementation has proved to be harmful. The truth is, management of GD does not work, because GD is not a disease.

The blood-glucose tests done in pregnancy to screen for gestational diabetes are questionable and based on faulty studies. Henci Goer, author of *"The Thinking Woman's Guide to a Better Birth,"* illustrates the problem with screening for gestational diabetes very clearly. The following quotation is taken from her article *Gestational Diabetes - The Emperor Has No Clothes;*

"The main rationale for current GD management is to reduce the incidence of birth injuries and cesarean section by reducing the incidence of macrosomia, [abnormally high birth weight.] The goal of reducing birth weight raises

philosophical problems. As with glucose values, doctors are defining deviation beyond an arbitrary point as inherently pathological. Moreover, can we justify manipulating the growth mechanism of a group of babies roughly 75 percent to 80 percent of whom will fall below the 90th percentile for weight if left alone?

"Philosophical considerations aside, we have little evidence that GD management succeeds. As mentioned above, macrosomia associates with maternal weight, age, race, parity, and male fetus.

"Santini and Ales report results from a national trial that occurred in the early 1980's when some doctors at Cornell University Medical Center screened women for GD routinely and others did not. No differences in perinatal mortality, morbidity, LGA or macrosomia rates were found between screened and unscreened populations, but women in the screened population were more likely to have primary cesarean sections (19 percent versus 12 percent), more clinic visits, more fetal surveillance tests, and more prenatal hospitalization."

~ Henci Goer

Gestational Diabetes, in my opinion, is a complete fabrication from the medical industry and something not worth worrying about if you are planning an unassisted birth. That's just my opinion, though, and if you do have concern, then additional information can be obtained on the subject.

To be clear, pre-existing diabetes, (Type I or II diabetes diagnosed before pregnancy,) is *not* a fabrication, and does have implications that can negatively affect maternal health and fetal development. Unlike gestational diabetes, true diabetes is disease with real implications and which requires a management strategy.

Problematic Swelling & Toxemia

Minor swelling does not indicate toxemia and poses no problems for mother or baby. (See the above section for minor swelling issues.) Aviva Romm describes problematic swelling as "swelling that is present all the time, swelling that leaves an impression on your leg a few seconds after you press on it, or swelling that particularly occurs in your face and hands that is visible the first thing in the morning." These types of swelling may indicate toxemia, especially if accompanied with high blood pressure, a general feeling of unwellness, nausea past the first trimester, headaches, blurry vision, low blood sugar, abdominal pain, lack of appetite, an underweight baby, and protein in the urine.

"Inadequate nutrition is the common denominator in toxemia."

~Aviva Romm

Toxemia is also often called pre-eclampsia, can be serious and shouldn't be overlooked if it develops. The best mode of action here is prevention. I will offer some advice on preventative methods so that toxemia does not develop. If it does develop, my suggestion is consult a midwife or an experienced natural health practitioner.

Toxemia almost always develops because of malnutrition, and can be prevented in almost all cases by excellent self-care, including eating nutritious foods, drinking plenty of nourishing "pregnancy tonic" teas and infusions, getting lots of sun on your skin (for vitamin D,) eating plenty of protein, (at least 60 grams a day,) salting your food to taste with real sea salt, including traditional fats like butter in your diet, and eating as soon as you are hungry.

Poverty puts women at greater risk for toxemia due to lack of available high-quality foods. Teen mothers and women who tend to weight-loss-dieting & over-exercise are also at greater risk for the same reason.

Drink lots and lots of nettle and dandelion teas. By now you may have noticed that Nettle tea is a remedy for just about every issue in pregnancy, and it can be used as a preventative for toxemia, too. Drink 2 cups a day. Dandelion leaf and root are both helpful, as well as burdock root and yellow dock root, in helping the liver and kidneys to function optimally. Epsom or Dead Sea salt baths can also be helpful in providing the body with sufficient magnesium and helping to detoxify the body. Add one cup to a warm bath, soak for no more than 20 minutes, and then rinse off.

Well-nourished and healthy-feeling women are extremely unlikely to develop toxemia.

Premature Rupture of Membranes

If the amniotic sac ruptures more than one hour before the onset of labor, this is called "premature rupture of membranes" also known as PROM or the breaking of waters. There are preventative home treatments that can be employed to ensure a strong amniotic sac and to make the likelihood of PROM very slim. One such remedy is simply making sure to get enough vitamin C through dietary sources, or, if dietary vitamin C is not available, in the form of a vitamin C supplement.

Abnormal bacteria (such as BV), and abnormal pH of the vagina are also indicated in PROM. According to midwife Gail Hart, "*pH alone—the acid/alkaline level measured by nitrazine or litmus paper—is a marker for prematurity risk. Retrospective and prospective studies show that high vaginal pH (a low acid, or alkaline, state) is predictive of preterm labor and preterm rupture of membranes.*" A simple home test can indicate whether your vaginal pH is ideal. If it isn't, good bacteria are the key! Lactic acid is produced in the vagina by *Lactobacilli*. Re-colonizing the vagina with lactobacilli can be as simple as taking a probiotic supplement, eating more yogurt and fermented foods, or even applying plain yogurt externally to the vagina.

If your waters *do* break prematurely, there are some herbal remedies that can be helpful in preventing infection and, possibly even healing the amniotic sac.

Nettle and comfrey leaf infusions can both be helpful in re-sealing a ruptured amniotic sac. Drink up to a quart of a strong nettle leaf infusion every day. Comfrey can also be a great aid in healing.

Comfrey has come under scrutiny in recent years as certain alkaloids in the plant can cause liver damage. Wild comfrey (Symphytum officinalis,) has small white flowers and has these alkaloids concentrated throughout the plant, and should be avoided during pregnancy. Cultivated Comfrey, (Symphytum uplandica,) has purple flowers and was bred to reduce alkaloid content of the leaves. The larger, mature leaves are safe to use as an infusion during pregnancy, and can promote rapid healing,(of any part of the body, including the amniotic sac.) Avoid the roots, young shoots, and young leaves during pregnancy – only use the mature (older) leaves. (If you have a history of liver damage then it may be best to err on the side of caution and avoid comfrey entirely during pregnancy.)

If membranes rupture then daily use of echinacea tincture, 20 drops 2 or 3 times a day, can help to ward off infection, as can garlic and a diet rich in vitamin C.

If membranes rupture (fully) prematurely, do not heal, and you don't go into labor within a few days, Blue cohosh root can be used to induce contractions and begin labor. Blue cohosh should only be used if you are over 37 weeks pregnant and believe your baby is actually ready for birth. The dose, according to Susun Weed, is *"3-8 drops in a glass of warm water or tea..."* Weed recommends repeating the dose *"every half hour for several hours until contractions are regular. If labor is not underway in four hours, use a dropperful of the tincture under the tongue every hour for up to four more hours or until contractions are strong and consistent."*

Some Herbs to Avoid during Pregnancy

Herbs are powerful, and should be respected for their power. There are many herbs that, although they may be amazing allies at other times of life, are not suitable for use during pregnancy.

Pennyroyal, mugwort, angelica & dong quai, wild carrot seed, rue, tansy, juniper berries & root, tansy, cotton seed or root, asafetida, celery seed, black cohosh, & blue cohosh should all be strictly avoided during pregnancy as they can cause birth defects and spontaneous abortion. (Blue cohosh is used by some as a late pregnancy tonic but I wouldn't personally recommend using it until after the onset of labor.)

Many common cooking herbs, like parsley, nutmeg, sage, rosemary, horseradish, and basil, can be emmenagogues and should be avoided completely in the first few months of pregnancy by those with a likelihood of miscarriage, and used very sparingly otherwise. (An emmenagogue is an herb that brings on or increases menstruation. Not all emmenagogues will cause miscarriage, but still, care should be taken.) Other herbs to avoid during pregnancy include feverfew, lobelia, arnica, aloe, poke root, calamus, osha, shepherd's purse, wormwood, goldenseal, licorice root and yarrow. This is not a complete list, so always do your research if you are unsure as to whether an herb is safe to use during pregnancy.

Flower Essence Therapy during Pregnancy

I have had incredible experiences with the subtle healing power of flower essences, especially after the birth of my first daughter. Flower essences are, as described by Patricia Kaminski and Richard Katz, "subtle liquid extracts, generally taken in oral form... prepared from a sun infusion of either wildflowers or pristine garden blossoms in a bowl of water, which is further diluted and potentized." You can learn to craft your own flower essences, althoughalternatively you can find them for sale at many health food stores.

Flower essences are great allies during pregnancy, when emotional tension and imbalance can be exposed more clearly due to increased demands on the body. Flower essences can help balance emotional disparity and loosen emotional tension. They can transform fears, open hearts and minds, and inspire vibrant well-being. Rather than affecting our physical bodies, flower essences heal and nourish on a vibrational, emotional, and spiritual level, which can subsequently open the body to greater healing and nourishment.

Developing relationships with certain flowers in nature or in your garden has the same, if not a much greater effect on emotional and spiritual health as the bottled flower essences you can purchase or craft. Bottled flower essences can offer support, but if you do have the time to relate to flowers in nature, this is a more potent form of connecting with a flower's essence. Bottles flower essences are helpful, however, in that they can be used continually throughout the day with minimal effort.

The following descriptions of the benefits of different flower essences could apply to either the bottled essences that you can craft or purchase, or to developing a relationship with the flowers around you. There are as many flower essences as there are flowers, so obviously I couldn't include them all in this book. I will only include flower essences that I have found helpful for myself, or ones that seem to apply to specific physical, mental, emotional, and spiritual issues that might develop during pregnancy or childbirth. Of course, everyone's relationship to certain flowers will be unique, but there seem to be certain empirical energies that carry over from person to person.

Rose – Rose is one of humanity's most loved flowers. Rose flowers are the essence of open-hearted giving, love, and receptivity. Rose engages and uplifts the energy of the heart, providing enthusiasm for living and sharing one's gifts. Rose can remedy depression, lack of vitality, and inability to nourish and inspire oneself due to apathy.

Manzanita – Manzanita flower essence provides love for the body. It helps to ground one's presence in the physical body and brings joy and light to this experience. Manzanita can help those who experience eating disorders or extreme dislike of their bodies to accept physical nourishment joyously.

California Pitcher Plant – California Pitcher Plant flower essence carries a grounding, nourishing and vitalizing essence. This flower essence is indicated for listlessness, tiredness, mental & emotional fatigue, and weak digestion. It is also helpful for those who are afraid of their instinctual self and their innate bodily intelligence. I used California Pitcher Plant flower essence when I was experiencing iron-deficiency anemia in my second pregnancy, and found it to be very helpful.

Dogwood – Dogwood flowers are soft and graceful. They impart this essence, providing softness and ease; they help to relax and soften rigid, tense, and harsh qualities.

Pine – Pine is a very helpful flower essence for those who are prone to self-ridicule. Pine can help if you find that you blame yourself, criticize yourself, or feel guilty about your actions or thoughts. Pine flower essence can help to transform these immobilizing feelings into a positive self-image, where constructive criticism has a place, but it is not all-consuming.

Sagebrush – Sagebrush is my favorite flower essence. It is incredibly potent in its healing potential, and many people experience dramatic shifts in their life experience when they use Sagebrush. Sagebrush is clearing and very opening. It is about letting go – letting go of ideas, of beliefs, of perceptions of who we are or how we 'should' conduct our lives. It opens the emotional body to transformation by clearing any blockage or barrier. I feel like there was a radical shift in my emotional state after I started using Sagebrush. Sagebrush flower essence works very well in combination with other flower essences – I feel it amplifies the other flower essences by making the emotional body more receptive to change.

Aspen – Aspen flower essence can help us to let go of fear and anxiety around the "unknown." It helps us relax, providing confidence and trust that the wisdom of life will guide us. It gives us strength to meet the unknown, to overcome fears of the future, which can be very helpful when you are on your journey to birth.

Olive – I have found olive flower essence to be extremely helpful, especially in the post-partum period. Olive is indicated where there is extreme exhaustion and depletion of life-force. Olive flower essence helps to restore vitality and renew physical and emotional energy.

Cerato – Cerato flower essence is incredibly applicable to many issues surrounding pregnancy and childbirth. Cerato flowers inspire trust in our inner knowledge – our intuition. They inspire self-reliance rather than over-dependence on others for opinions and advice. Cerato helps us to overcome uncertainty and learn to listen to our inner voice. Patricia Kaminski and Richard Katz write that cerato helps in "developing trust in one's inner knowing; relying on the strength of one's inner guidance when choosing prenatal and natal care."

Self Heal – Self Heal flower essence helps us tap into our own healing potential, rather than relying on others for healing. True healing comes from within.

Dandelion – Dandelion flower essence brings ease, joy, and relaxation to those who tend to be very rigid and tense. Those who Dandelion can help lean towards a mentality that work must be hard to be effective. They are overachievers and "hard" workers.

Dandelion helps these people to realize that easy and free-flowing work can be even more effective than "hard" work. Dandelion helps people to get in touch with the needs of their bodies, and is especially proficient at releasing emotional tensions. This is another of my favorite flower essences.

Oak – Oak flower essence is for the "hero." It is for the provider. Oak helps mothers who have lots of responsibilities, who tend put others needs before their own. Oak is an incredibly strong and powerful tree, but it is also rigid. It is so rigid that it cannot bend, and so it breaks if too much weight is put upon it. Oak carries the message that it is ok to let go – it is ok to bend and be flexible. Sometimes, the strongest trees are the ones who can bend. Oak helps mothers learn the ability to let go of perceived responsibilities, or at least to pay attention to their own needs rather than always focusing on the needs of others.

Cayenne – The flowers of Cayenne pepper can be extremely helpful for eliminating stagnation. Cayenne provides a fiery essence that imparts movement and momentum. If you are feeling stuck or stagnant, indecisive or immobile, cayenne can be of great help.

Agrimony & Black Eyed Susan – Both Agrimony and Black Eyed Susan flowers are indicated when there is denial of pain, fear, or true feelings. These essences help you to acknowledge inner truths and desires – they help to unmask hidden feelings.

Penstemon – Penstemon flowers impart strength – They provide the ability to meet challenge, to overcome adversity, and to thrive in even the harshest conditions. Penstemon can help to provide self confidence and trust in your body's strength and innate ability to give birth in any environment.

Willow – Willow is very helpful for releasing bitterness and resentment, and for taking responsibility for yourself. Willow imparts the ability to forgive, let go, and go with the flow of life. Willow flower essence imparts flexibility and grace. Think of willow – she is beautiful, graceful, magical; she bends gracefully and does not break, even in the harshest winds & she can root herself easily in new places

& new situations – this is the gift of willow's flower essence.

Borage – Borage flower essence provides courage, joy, and optimism. Borage can help lift your spirit, or provide relief from gloom, discouragement, or heavy-heartedness.

Chamomile – Chamomile flower essence provides calm and serenity. It can help to release emotional tension, especially in the solar-plexus.

Indian Pink –Indian Pink flower essence helped me to feel centered and grounded during times of high activity after the birth of my first child. This was a huge transition, one I was unprepared for, and I remember always telling my mate that I felt "behind." I felt like there was so much to do and no time to get any of it done! Indian Pink helped incredibly – I noticed a huge difference in my emotional state and was able to handle a number of tasks simultaneously while caring for an infant in a much more composed manor!

Angelica – Angelica flower essence provides spiritual guidance & protection. It instills a sense of faith in life and in your safety in any situation. It can be used for to face and overcome fear of giving birth, or fear of death in childbirth.

Mariposa Lily – Most lilies carry a feminine essence. Mariposa lily is specific to the "mother" aspect of the feminine archetype. Mariposa lily can be used to heal the mother-child relationship; it helps connect us with the mother earth, to our own mothers, and to ourselves as mothers.

Pink Yarrow – Pink Yarrow flower essence can be helpful for mothers who are sensitive to cultural or familial negativity around birth. This essence is helpful for women who are oversensitive to others fears and negative stories of birth. Pink yarrow lets you sort through and find out what are your own thoughts and feelings about birth, rather than the thoughts, feelings, and stories of others.

Five-Flower Formula or Rescue Remedy – These formulas are designed to bring immediate calm, stress relief, and the ability to relax and let go of hysteria or deep fears. These formulas both contain Clematis, Cherry Plum, Impatiens, Rock Rose, and Star of Bethlehem flower essences. They can help in traumatic situations and during times of profound transition.

If you are using bottled flower essences, a dose is four drops under the tongue four times a day, or four drops in a glass of pure water sipped throughout the day. Flower essences can also be applied topically, on the wrists or forehead or any part of the body. Flower essences are completely, utterly safe.

> *"To comprehend fully the incredible love, intelligence, vital life force and healing energy of the herbs and plants, we need to enter into resonance with them. To learn the many secrets of the plants, we need to learn their language. To learn the language of the plants, we need to listen deeply, with an open, humble, and grateful heart."*
>
> *~Gail Faith Edwards*

Movement & Rest

This chapter is very simple. When it comes to movement and rest, your body has needs. Sometimes you are tired, drained, and worn out. When this happens: rest, retreat, and sleep. When this happens, turn off the lights, the phone, the computer – turn off your thoughts about what needs to be done. Let yourself let it go, for the sake of your well-being. Warm up a cup of herbal tea, or some nourishing leftovers, on the stove. Sit by the fire or rest on the couch, and feel your body relax. Step outside. Walk to your favorite tree, or bench, and sit and take a deep breath. These are all great ways to nourish your body in preparation for childbirth.

Other times, your energy rises and you feel abundant. You feel excited and passionate! When this happens: move, create, explore. Don't let yourself be cooped up inside for too long – this energy is too big for that! It needs to spread out! Make passionate love, or go for a long meandering walk. Explore somewhere you have never been before. Work in the garden or do some outdoor chores. These are all wonderful ways to tone your body in preparation for childbirth.

There is a balance to this dance – too much movement and you can deplete yourself in one way. Too much rest, and you can deplete yourself in another way. Too much movement without taking the time to rest and nurture can cause malnourishment, tension, and irritability. Too much rest without taking the time to move around a bit creates stagnation – your organs, muscles, and the systems of your body start to move more slowly and function less than optimally.

Once you have learned to listen to and act upon the cues of your body, recognizing and acting upon the cues of rest and movement becomes much easier. Maintaining the balance becomes innate. You are neither overworked and depleted, nor stagnant and apathetic – rather, you are both fulfilled and rested in every moment.

There is a little more to it, I suppose, but it is still quite simple:

Regaining balance can be more difficult than *maintaining* balance. If an imbalance occurs in one of these areas, it might take a bit of a push – a conscious effort on your part – to regain balance. If, for example, you are prone to a very sedentary lifestyle, your muscles may not be toned enough to make regular healthy movement as effortless as it should be; it may take a bit of effort to go for a walk, weed a row in the garden, or move in some other beneficial way. If this is the case, do not push yourself, but learn to recognize your body's needs for healthy movement and act on those needs when they arise.

On the other hand, if you are prone to too much movement – excessive doing and creating and accomplishing without taking care of your body's basic needs for rest and food, then it may be difficult to let go, once in a while, and rest. There may be mental and emotional barriers to letting yourself rest that are hard to let go of. The truth is that in letting these belief barriers go, you will not harm yourself, and you will probably not miss out on anything. By taking the time to nourish yourself, you will become more capable, more effective, and more efficient. If this is the case for you, learn to recognize your body's need for rest and nourishment, and learn to let go of the belief barriers that keep you from acting upon these needs.

No two people are the same when it comes to these needs. There is not an all-encompassing formula for the human body that says 50% rest and 50% movement is the optimal ratio to create a balanced human. Everyone is different – some drastically different. Perhaps the average person needs half rest and half movement, but some will need mostly movement and little rest, or mostly rest and little movement. No one can tell you what balance of rest and movement is right for you – only you can know through your honest intuitive insight into your own body's needs.

Making Love: Making love is an amazing and balanced form of movement. There are differing traditional customs when it comes to having sex during pregnancy. Some cultures completely abstain, some 'accept,' and some encourage sex.

Love making has been shown to have numerous benefits for pregnant women. Besides strengthening and toning the leg and pelvic muscles which helps prepare the body for birth, making love encourages oxytocin, the "hormone of love," which plays an important role in labor, and helps to soften the cervix. Many women report going into labor just after making love.

There are many corresponding aspects between love-making and birth – many of the same hormones are required, and because of this, making love is a good way to practice, so to speak, for the birth process.

You can notice, while making love, if you have any inhibitions – you can notice what you feel about your body, and if you have thoughts that get in the way of pleasure. You can notice the atmosphere – what setting makes you most comfortable? In what setting so you feel the least inhibited?

When you feel uninhibited and passionate while making love, this is because your hormones are functioning optimally. The setting that lets you 'let go' while making love will also let you 'let go' during labor. This setting, of course, is different for everyone, but there seems to be some general overlap in most cases: non-observation, dim lighting, and intimacy.

Cultural Fear

*"The most fundamental difference between our ancient tribal
sisters and modern birthing women is that our ancestors
fully trusted their bodies to birth easily and effortlessly."*

~*Veronika Sophia Robinson*

The fear-based image of birth that is so prevalent in mainstream North American culture leads many people to believe that birth is inherently dangerous. Women are too often convinced that when they become pregnant and go into labor, they will experience excruciating pain and be in utter peril. They are led to believe that constant monitoring is necessary in order to ensure their and their baby's safety. Birth is still portrayed in movies and TV shows as something very complicated, requiring IV anesthetics and sterile gloves.

This is not an honest representation of birth!

Although I and many others know that birth is an innate biological process, this knowledge is not accessible to many men and women.

Many people view birth as dangerous, and because this is their view, they will of course take it upon themselves to protect or correct loved ones who make unconventional birth choices. All too often I hear stories from pregnant women planning unassisted births that illustrate this.

Recently I came across a question on a popular unassisted birthing website from a woman *whoseown father and brother* had threatened to come and *force* her to go to the hospital once she started labor. This woman was asking for advice from others on the website to find out if they had experience with this sort of violent threat. Many who answered had similar stories to tell.

I hear another similar story,repeated over and over with a bit of variation each time - from many of the mothers who I meet; always the same story: They tell me that they had a very strong desire to have an unassisted birth, or even just a home birth, but that their husband/partner wouldn't even consider the idea, and so they ended up planning a hospital birth instead. Honestly, I feel like there is no place for this when it comes to birth. The birth plan should be left entirely to the birthing mother, and should be completely respected by the father or partner to the best of their ability. Although suggestions are always helpful and expressions of fear or concern are *necessary*, the ultimate choice of where and how to give birth is best left to the woman who'll actually be doing the birthing! The mother knows what is right for her baby, her body, and her birth.

Luckily, I did not experience this sort of overt hostility from family members and friends when they found out about my plans to birth without assistance. I did, however, experience a whole lot of fear and anxiety coming from my family.

Eventually, most of my family became aware that I did not plan to seek out a midwife or a physician for my prenatal care and birth. Many found this to be a serious issue of safety. I was told often that I was putting my baby's life in danger. I was told that I was irresponsible. I was told that I would have to hire a midwife. I was told that I could die.

I am so grateful for the support I found, through books, forums, birth stories, and statistics. They confirmed that my intuition was probably not going haywire, like my family seemed to think. I am also infinitely grateful for the support of Joey, my partner. Without those written resources and Joey's unwavering confidence and support, I may have finally given in to fear. I may have sought a midwife. I may have invited her into our tiny, intimate one-room log cabin on that snowy day in March when my daughter chose to make her appearance. That day, Peacy's birth day, was the most beautiful, monumental, empowering, intimate, and intense few hours I had ever experienced up to that point in my life. Looking back, I cannot imagine someone else in that space – that sacred, potent birthing space. I am so, so, so glad that I stayed true to my intuition and did not give in to fear.

So, how do you navigate a culture so bent on a belief that birth is dangerous? How do you deal with family members who agonize and worry over your birth choice, and even threaten to force you to choose differently? There are a few tactics.

One way, which is quite simple and sheepishly alluring, is to inform your family that you've become pregnant when you are already at about four or five months gestation. Wear loose clothing, keep quiet, and enjoy this little secret between you and your partner. I found that my family really started to agonize when I was around 7 or 8 months pregnant. If you keep the baby a secret for long enough, he or she will be earthside before anyone even has a chance to worry! Sure… they may wonder why you're suddenly becoming nauseous at the thought of scrambled eggs when you once loved them, and yeah… it's hard to keep a secret from your own mother, the woman who gave birth to you and knows you better than anyone. But, if you feel like your family or others in your life may be overtly unsupportive of or hostile to your birth choice, then it is certainly within your right to keep a little distance for a few months. Simple, straightforward, and effective.

If this last option is not your cup of tea, I totally understand. I couldn't wait to tell my family I was pregnant! I love them and wanted nothing more than to share this bit of joy with them! We may live different lifestyles and make different choices, but the idea of cutting my family out of my life or omitting this joyous news from them wasn't something I considered in my pregnancies, and isn't something I would consider in the future.

The true way to navigate this culture is with strength and confidence. Know your body, know your truth, and do not be afraid to express it. If there are people in your life who are agonizing over you, then know it is their own fear that they face, and not your responsibility to relieve them of this anxiety. If you are being told negative birth story after negative birth story by friends, then simply let your friends know that you don't need that kind of negativity. Let them know that you have made your choice, that you trust your body, and that the fear-based view of birth is not the truth of birth. You don't need to be insensitive – it is easy to experience birth as dangerous when that is your belief; the people who share these stories with you probably legitimately care about you and are trying to help you in the only way they know how. At the same time, if people are threatening you, harassing you, or crossing your boundaries in any way, then do not be afraid to cut them out of your life for the time being.

Due Dates & Patience

I love picking berries in the summer. Right now our black raspberries are almost ripe! When you find a ripe raspberry and pluck it from the cane, it falls away effortlessly, and the sweet, juicy summer goodness melts in your mouth. The raspberries that aren't quite ripe still hold to the cane when tugged; if these are picked anyhow, they will never be as juicy or as sweet as the berries which are left to mature in their own time.

Have you ever picked the seed-head of a dandelion and blown on it? It can be so satisfying find the ripe ones! When blown on, the seeds partreadily from the stalk, floating gracefully down to their new homes. Then there are the seeds which, even though they appear full and ripe, are just not quite ready to part with the stalk. No matter how hard you blow, they hold on tight! They have an innate intelligence – they know just the right time to let go to ensure that they have the resilience to face the world on their own.

We hold that intelligence too, as do our babies. Just as the fruit will not part from the bush until it is ready – just as the seed waits, so do our babies. They have so much work to do in readying themselves for the outside world, and if we ask to come before their time through induction of any sort, even a day or a minute missed in the womb could be too much!

Recent findings indicate that the initiation of full-term labor is triggered by the release of a protein from the lungs of the fetus. This protein is essential for normal extra-uterine breathing, and its release initiates a cascade of biological reactions which finally result in labor. Thus, looking more closely at our biology and chemistry shows us what we already intuitively know; our babies know when they are ready to be born – everything happens in its own time. Our babies make the spark that fuels the fire of our labor when they are ready for life outside the womb.

An average human gestation is around 282 days, or ten lunar cycles, but that average can swing about 3 weeks in either direction. Due date estimation is definitely not an exact science. Even if you know the exact moment that your baby was conceived, each baby develops at his or her own pace, and an accurate prediction of your due date based on the length of an average human gestation is really not realistic! Due dates are a nice estimate, but they are not something to be taken too seriously. Intuition is a better tool in determining when your baby will come earthside.

Putting too much stock in a due date can cause stress. I miscalculated the due dates of my first two children. I knew the date of their conception, and so I assumed I would just calculate 40 weeks from there and that would give me my due date. Little did I know that when calculating from conception, you only need to count ahead by 38 weeks! Based on my *mis*calculations, Peacy came three weeks early, and Micah came 'early' by a little under two weeks. Really, they weren't early at all!

When I became pregnant with Ahmik, my third child, I calculated 40 weeks from the first day of my last period – the standard due date calculation. January 6th. Well, January 6th came, and then went. Even though in my heart I know babies are born in their own time, I still felt stressed. I knew she was close, but the thought of having passed my due date made me wonder – how long would I be waiting? I had prepared to give birth in early January…. Would I be waiting until February?? I didn't feel prepared to wait that long – not because I was worried for her health or for mine, but because I had made all the necessary preparations for her birth, and I just felt impatient! Ahmik came on January 15th – the perfect day.

There is plenty of misleading and outdated information prevalent in our culture around "overdue" or "postterm" babies. Stillbirth, placental failure, and macrosomia are some of the fears that come up for us because of this misinformation. Luckily, there is evidence now that postterm babies are actually better suited for extrauterine life – they score higher on Apgar tests and are generally better able to latch on and thrive. So, if you are past your due date, know that your baby is probably just patiently waiting until they are full and ready for the best possible start they can get in life!

Placental failure has been shown to be a myth. The idea that a placenta ages and is at the point of failure near 40 weeks gestation comes from a misunderstanding of the placenta. The placenta does undergo noticeable changes as pregnancy progresses, particularly in the structure of the villi, but it does not age nor is it nearing the end of its functionality at term. Rather, the placenta *matures* and actually *increases in efficiency*, becoming more effective in the conduction of oxygen from mother to child as pregnancy progresses! The following excerpts, which detail this point, are taken from a peer-reviewed article by Harold Fox from the University of Manchester. *"It has often been implied that this changing appearance [of the villi of the placenta] is an aging process, but it is now recognized that this temporal variability in villous appearances reflects the continual development and branching of the villous tree... The processes of maturation of the villous tree results in a predominant villous form that is optimally adapted for materno-fetal transfer diffusion mechanisms... A review of the available evidence indicates that the placenta does not undergo a true aging change during pregnancy. There is, in fact, no logical reason for believing that the placenta, which is a fetal organ, should age while the other fetal organs do not: the situation in which an individual organ ages within an organism that is not aged is one which does not occur in any biological system."*

When we look at the evidence, there is no scientific basis to support induction of postterm babies. The opinion that carrying a child beyond 41 weeks carries inherent risks comes from a study which was conducted in 1958. This study is well outdated. More recent studies show that there is hardly any increased risk at all from 41 weeks to 42 weeks – a 0.1% increase in the chance of stillbirth – and there is *no reason to suspect* that this increase is due to carrying into the 42nd week.

According to Gail Hart, there is a chance that a baby carried past 43 weeks could suffer postmaturity syndrome, but she cites that *"less than 90%"* of babies born after 43 weeks will show any signs at all, meaning that the vast majority of babies born in the late range of a normal pregnancy were actually not "late" at all, but just on time. My guess is that, in the small percentage (less than 10%) of babies born after 43 weeks who *did* show signs of postmaturity syndrome, there was some sort of emotional or psychological blockage, such as fear, which prevented the initiation of the natural orchestration of labor. (More on that in Part III, Chapter 2.)

Induction, whether via the hospital or via home/herbal means, carries inherent risks. It is better that we trust our bodies and our babies to know their time. If something truly feels amiss, then induction, (herbal or otherwise,) might be the best option, but in the vast majority of pregnancies the complications associated with premature induction are dangerous, while the alternative – patience – is not.

> *"Much of our prenatal care is based on bringing babies to birth "in a timely fashion"—neither too early nor too late. But our understanding of "timely" is clouded, and some of our methods are self-defeating. By intervening in the natural timing of birth, we sometimes exacerbate the problems or create entirely new ones."*
>
> ~Gail Hart

Less talked about in our culture are babies who go well beyond the 43 week mark and are born strong and healthy. In a normal unhindered pregnancy, many women go to 44 weeks, some even to 45. According to a recent study, there is a normal, healthy 37 day variation in the length of human gestation. That would put the end of the 'normal' range at 42 weeks and 6 days, or almost 43 weeks. However, that study only followed 130 participants, and the study did not exclude pregnancies which ended in induction or cesarean! Rather, they *"accounted for events that artificially shorten the natural length of gestation."* But how could they know how long those pregnancies would have gone without intervention? If a more conclusive study were undertaken with a large and diverse population of subjects, where the subjects were left unhindered and labor was left to initiate spontaneously, I am willing to bet that the natural variation in gestational length would be much greater.

Studies have found a few factors which can influence the length of gestation; women who are older tend to carry longer, as do women who were born with a higher birth weight. Hormones also play a role. According to a 2013 study, *"pregnancies with a rapid progesterone rise were longer than those with delayed rise."*

Another phenomenon, knows as embryonic diapause or delayed implantation, could also be a factor. An embryo develops on its own up to a certain point before being implanted in the uterus. The point at which the embryo implants is called the "blastocyst stage." If an embryo reaches this stage and finds an unreceptive uterus, the embryo can essentially enter hibernation – it will not develop further and and pregnancy will be suspended. Embryonic diapause is a common response in many mammals, including marsupials, rodents, and carnivores, to environmental stressors such as lack of food, time of year, and drought. Once conditions are favorable, these mammals are able to resume pregnancy, thus timing the birth of their babies for a more suitable time when survival is more likely.

Until recently, embryonic diapause was thought to be a trait of only a small handful of mammals. However, new studies may indicate that embryonic diapause is innate in *all* mammals, including humans. *"If proven, the existence of human embryo diapause could question the adequacy of common gynecological practices, such as the estimation of the gestational age based on the last menstrual cycle or the stimulation of parturition. This hypothesis, if confirmed, would have a great impact on human reproductive medicine... Accordingly, common obstetric definitions, such as "foetus small for gestational age" or "prolonged pregnancy" may need to be revised."*

There are also uncommon cases of abnormal pregnancies, caused by environmental stressors and hormonal imbalances, which can go much longer than 44-45 weeks. This phenomenon is not well-recognized in the sphere of western medicine, but it does happen, and maybe more often than we are aware of.

There are little or no human studies documenting such pregnancies, and there is not even any good terminology to describe them! Cultural terms have been designated out of necessity – cryptic pregnancy is one such term, but it is misleading and unclear, because it can refer to a pregnancy in which a woman does not know she is pregnant, or to a pregnancy in which a woman's body does not fully recognize the pregnancy hormonally, but intuitively she knows she is pregnant. The latter of these types of pregnancy can last quite a long time – many months over the normal length of gestation – and are characterized by continued menstrual cycles during gestation, abnormally slow fetal weight gain, and negative pregnancy tests (both urine and blood tests, due to lack of hCG hormone in mother's system.) However, if taken, fetal heart tones will be found, confirming the pregnancy is genuine and not a "phantom pregnancy."

Because there is very little known about these types of pregnancies, I cannot elaborate much on them. What I have learned about them is from friends and second-hand accounts. In the future hopefully there will be more acceptance of and interest in this phenomenon from people who have the means to shed more light on it, but in the meantime what we *can* know is that there is so much we *don't* know! In that regard, trusting our bodies to carry our ancestral wisdom is more important than ever.

Although we may think we understand quite a lot about human reproduction, there is so much left undiscovered, and so much that is really beyond the realm of discovery. If our beliefs as a society dictate that intervention in the natural process of birth is necessary on a regular basis, my feeling is that those beliefs are seriously lacking and should be thoroughly questioned.

It is exciting to calculate a due date and envision life with a new child at that time, but setting too much store in it can cause unnecessary stress. Our children have the enormous pleasure of choosing their own birthdays. If left unhindered, they will choose the perfect day to enter the world.

Equipment for Freebirth

At some point during your pregnancy, the reality of your baby's approaching birthday might seem a bit more tangible. When this happens, you might find yourself wondering what you will need to do and collect to prepare for that day, and for the immediate post-partum period.

Here's what I did in preparation for my daughter's birth:

1.) Made sure we had a home to live in that we could heat. (Previously this had not been the case.)

2.) Relocated five or six big towels from my father's house to our new heat-efficient log cabin. (Purchasing towels would have been an equally valid option, except that there were about 100 towels in my dad's house, and I thought I could put a few of them to good use by giving birth on them.)

3.) Bought a bag of dried Shepherd's Purse herb for Joey to make into an infusion once labor began. (In retrospect, a tincture of Shepherd's Purse would have been a much better choice.)

4.) Made curtains for our windows.

That's about it...

As soon as I put the curtains up in the windows, I went into labor with my daughter.

When Peacy, my daughter, was 16 months old, we met a family in another state and decided to move to live with them. We had been looking for community for quite a while. We moved to their farm where we started to build a small cabin to live in. I was about 5 months pregnant with my son at the time. We finished building the cabin a month or so before I went into labor with my son, Micah.

I felt very assured during Micah's pregnancy that my body would act perfectly, and that there was little I needed to 'do' other than keep myself feeling nourished. Here's what I did in preparation for my son's birth:

1.) Made sure we had some clean towels on hand.

2.) Sewed curtains for our new cabin's windows.

Interestingly, a day or two after I put up the final curtain in our cabin, I went into labor with Micah.

Three years later, with another little one about to pop out, I was sewing curtains yet again. We had moved again, and had lived happily in this new house for almost two years with curtain-less windows. Now the windows seemed like big black holes, staring at me after sunset. This house seemed to have about a million windows, too. I covered all the ones I could, and about a week and a half later, my daughter was born.

The curtains, in all three cases, provided a sense of protection and completion – a "go-ahead" to give birth.

In regard to birth preparation, mama hormones will really kick in at a certain point –the "nesting" impulse. It is a common phenomenon. Women nearing their last month of pregnancy will feel an impulse to stay close to home and prepare their home thoroughly for the coming baby.

In regard tobirth gear, heavyequipment is really not necessary. A birth pool isn't necessary. A special instrument to cut the umbilical cord is not necessary. Bed liners aren't necessary. Curtains aren't necessary... *unless they are*. Birth equipment is not an essential component in giving birth. What is essential is that the mother feels safe and comfortable in her birthing space – that she feels ready, and sometimes that means having certain things on hand. For me, that apparently required sewing curtains to cover my windows for each of my three labors. That way I didn't feel like my neighbors would be peeping through. Honestly, when birth rolled around I didn't think at all about the windows – some of the curtains even stayed open – but it helped me feel ready in the weeks & days preceding my births, and so however odd it seemed, it *was* necessary. For others, that may mean other things need to fall into place; some mothers may feel comfortable only once they've purchased some "blue pads" or plastic bed-liners to protect a mattress from blood and birth fluid. You would be amazed at the body's capacity to hold back when you feel nervous or apprehensive – imagine trying to keep bloody mucus and birth waters off the rug as your baby is crowning!

In that regard, it may be helpful to prepare some things that you can labor over – a few towels or some old sheets, or invest in a bed liner so that you can labor in bed without worrying about staining your mattress.

If you want a water birth, then make sure you have a very spacious bath tub, or rent a birthing pool.

Some herbs can be helpful during labor or some, like shepherd's purse, may be helpful to have on hand immediately after the birth. (I will discuss herbs for childbirth in Part IV of this book.) Deciding if you want to have herbs on hand, and which herbs you'll want, is a good thing to consider a good few months before giving birth. Read through the chapter on herbs for childbirth, and see if any call your name.

If you are making your own herbal medicines, many plants can only be gathered fresh in the spring and summer. If you plan to make tinctures from purchased dried herbs, then you'll need to start making the tinctures at least eight weeks, if not much longer, before your estimated due date. (Many babies come a week or two earlier than expected.) If you plan to purchase ready-made tinctures, do this at least a month or two before your estimated due date, just in case of an early baby.

Some parents choose to take an Infant cardio-pulmonary resuscitation, (Infant CPR,) or neonatal resurrection, (NRP,) class at their local hospital. This will prepare you in case your infant is asphyxiated after birth and cannot be revived through other methods such as massage or the sound of your voice. (Infants are born severely asphyxiated in about 1% of births in the United States, for a variety of reasons, many of which are caused by medical intervention.)

There are also some materials that I found very helpful right after birth. I used a canning basin to catch the placenta when it came out. That's just what we had on hand. You can birth the placenta anywhere, but it's nice to have somewhere to put it afterwards. A big bowl, a basin, or a towel to wrap it in are all good options.

After giving birth, you'll bleed for anywhere from a few days to a week. The flow will be similar to the flow of a regular period. After giving birth, you'll want cloth menstrual pads, not tampons, to catch your blood. I prefer re-usable cotton menstrual pads for a few reasons: they feel softer and gentler, they are not bleached and do not contain other chemicals like disposable menstrual pads often do, I enjoy washing them, and they are reusable and better for the health of the earth. Whichever type of pads you choose, make sure you have some on hand for after the birth.

As far as equipment for your newborn baby, very little is needed. A newborn only has one true need: you. You keep him or her warm, you provide his or her nourishment – as long as you are warm and nourished, than s/he will be too. However, I did find that four or five baby blankets, a sling/infant baby wrap, and a good number of cloth diapers and a few diaper covers were very, very helpful after my children were born.

The most important factor, and the common denominator in all childbirth preparation, is to learn listen to and follow your intuition. Learn to trust and act upon the cues of your inner voice. This will not only help you to nourish yourself and prepare your home in the unique way that is essential to your unique body and baby, but it will also prepare you to listen to that same inner wisdom during the birth process itself.

PART III:

A Personal Choice

Birth is a Mirror

*"The people we are in relationship with are always a
mirror, reflecting our own beliefs, and simultaneously we are
mirrors, reflecting their beliefs. So... relationship is one of
the most powerful tools for growth.... If we look honestly at
our relationships, we can see so much about how we have
created them."*

~ Shakti Gawain

Relationships of any kind are always reflections of our beliefs. We depend on belief systems to function, and until something new is integrated into our belief system, it is often hard or impossible to experience that thing. A newborn has not yet developed a belief system. Because of this, a newborn's reality is very different from a child's, or an adult's. Things are integrated one by one, and slowly the newborn's reality begins to shift until it is formed into a functional, or dysfunctional, adult reality.

Here is an example of how our beliefs can shape our experience: if a woman holds a belief that men are inherently cruel, then she could be in a relationship with the most caring, loving, and kind man in the world and still perceive him as cruel. Beliefs are structured so that if you hold on to a belief, you can apply it to your experience as a whole, and no matter what you're experiencing, you will perceive it through the filter of that belief.

In this way, we create our realities through our beliefs; or, rather, a more accurate way of saying this would be that our beliefs limit our realities.

Our experience of birth depends greatly on our ideas and preconceptions about birth, and in this way, birth reflects our beliefs back to us. Birth is a mirror.

If you believe birth is unsafe, then you will experience birth as unsafe. If you believe birth is sacred, then you will experience a sacred birth. If you believe birth requires medical intervention, then medical intervention will probably be required at your birth. If you believe birth is an inborn function of your body, then you will experience it as so.

In many ways, you have the ability to create your reality through your thoughts and beliefs, and awareness of this capability has the potential to be very liberating. Some people have a name for this; they call it the "law of attraction." Awareness of this is a powerful tool for self-growth and change, but I believe people often take this too far, or misinterpret it entirely.

Just because a negative image or a fear or a thought arises does not mean you need to worry. It does not mean you have done something wrong and that your birth will follow the path of that negative thought just because it popped into your head. The truth is, thoughts happen. Thoughts about death, about pain, about scary situations – they all happen, and just because these thoughts happen does not mean your life will follow their course. A thought is different than a belief – beliefs are deeply held and limit our perception, while thoughts are generally passing and are a part of our perception.

When negative thoughts about birth arise, it is an opportunity to look deeper – what is your true belief about birth, or, even deeper, what is underneath those beliefs? What does your innate bodily wisdom convey? Instead of trying to make a negative thought disappear, really explore the thought. Where did it come from? Is it actually true for you? What *is* your true knowing, and is the thought congruous with that knowing, or is it just a thought? You will find your own answer.

Sure, affirmations have their place. It's nice to make drawings or collages or have a vision board or an altar that display positive birth images – these are beautiful and inspiring exercises, but I don't believe these exercises are necessary in order to have a beautiful birth, the same as it is not necessary to dispel negative thoughts about birth that may appear.

> *"Continually trying to look on the bright side interferes with our finding the wisdom that lies in the fruitful darkness. Continually striving upward toward the light means we never grow downward into our own feet, never become firmly rooted on the earth, never explore the darkness within and around us, a darkness without whose existence the light would have no meaning."*
>
> *~Stephen Buhner*

During my pregnancies, I had thoughts of death. I had thoughts and worries that my births would be slow or painful. But always underneath those thoughts was my truth – my inner knowing that birth is what my body is designed to do – that birth is innate – inerrant – encoded in my cellular memory. When I looked deeper, (and sometimes I had to look very deep,) I found all the courage and trust that I needed, and any negative thoughts became extraneous happenings rather than all-important life-altering phenomena that they are sometimes made out to be.

Fearful thoughts happen for all kinds of reasons – maybe you heard a birth story or read a book or saw a movie that inspired the thoughts. These thoughts don't hold any power over your birth experience – what holds the power is that deep, ancestral bodily knowing that lies inside of you – that giving birth is inherent in your bones – in your muscles – in your heart and soul. What does your body tell you about birth? This is the inner knowing that affects the true outcome of our birthing experiences. Our deeper expectations of birth are what shape our birth experience.

Why Do Complications Occur?

"The majority of problems in birth — both now and in the past — can be traced to three main causes: poverty, unnecessary medical intervention, and fear which triggers the fight/flight response and shuts down labor. Despite what most people believe, the act of birth itself is not dangerous, but our cultural beliefs and practices can make it so."

~*Laura Shanley, author of "Unassisted Childbirth"*

Why do complications occur during labor? If childbirth is inherently safe and effortless, why do so many women experience traumatic births and need medical intervention?

There are four main reasons that complications occur in childbirth. Laura Shanley cites three of these often in her writings and talks. These reasons are poverty, medical intervention, and fear. The fourth reason that complications occur during birth occurs when a birthing mother is out of touch with her body and her intuition.

Poverty & Malnutrition – Living in poverty prevents women from obtaining optimal nourishment during pregnancy. Without access to nutritious foods, women become malnourished and often develop complications.

If you look at a graph displaying maternal mortality rate compared with the economic status of the mothers in question, you can see an astronomical decline in maternal mortality as economic status rises. This is because poverty and low economic status limit the choices that mothers have when it comes to prenatal care and nourishment.

Today, many mothers, children, and pregnant women live in food-insecure homes and are forced to make food choices which do not support their health. Much of the time, inexpensive foods like grains and beans won't provide enough nutrients to support a healthy pregnancy. If pasture-raised meats, fresh vegetables, fish, fruit, eggs, healthy fats like butter or coconut oil, and grass-fed dairy are added to this diet, malnutrition is much less likely, but these types of foods are usually much more expensive, and often not an option for very low-income families.

Poverty is also often congruous with a poor living environment. Women in poverty often live in cities with high levels of air pollution and little access to natural places. Access to clean air, clean water, and natural beauty are often much overlooked elements needed to support a healthy pregnancy.

Working long hours throughout pregnancy, often without sufficient food and rest breaks, is often necessary for women of low economic status. This can put a huge stress on the body and manifest as malnutrition, extreme fatigue, or general ill-health.

This absolutely does not mean that women without economic means will develop complications. Clearly for many women around the world, this is not true. What it means is that poverty is a major factor to consider if you are searching for the origin of a pregnancy or birth complication.

Women who have the means to afford plenty of nutritious foods, who drink clean, unpolluted water, and who have access to natural places and clean air will likely not develop complications in pregnancy or experience difficulty giving birth due to malnutrition or ill-health. If these women experience birth complications, it is more likely because of medical intervention or fear.

Medical Intervention – Medical intervention causes complications by interfering with the mother's natural instincts and hindering the birth process. Medical intervention can slow or stop the birth process, causing stress or pain, which all too often results in fetal distress or unnecessary C-sections.

Medical intervention can take many forms, from the subtle to the extreme. Subtle intervention involves suggesting certain birth positions to the mother, timing of contractions, asking the mother to relay her experience, or routine cervical checks. These interventions require the mother to come out of her birthing bubble, so to speak, and enter into the world of medical observation and monitoring. It breaks up the natural flow of birth.

More extreme interventions, like dilation checks without permission, use of Pitocin, anesthetics, and other labor drugs, or overt manipulation or degradation of the birthing mother can have extreme consequences, including physical or emotional trauma and postpartum depression.

If left unhindered, a woman's' cervical dilation can go from 3 centimeters to a full 10 centimeters in a matter of minutes, but if during that time she was laying on her back being "checked," or being asked to try a certain position, or being asked questions or listening to her husband count the seconds between each contraction, this quick progression of labor may not be allowed to occur. If, during the time that this quick cervical dilation might have occurred, the woman was experiencing degradation, birth rape, use of drugs or other extreme medical interventions, birth might never be allowed to progress.

*"A woman does not need busyness around her, and she
certainly doesn't need to be told how to breathe or push.
Birth is instinctive and if left alone, a woman will
automatically do these things."*

~Veronika Sophia Robinson

Birth happens best in quiet, calm locations, with dim lighting, little talking, and little disturbance of the laboring mother. If a birthing woman needs assistance, she will ask for it. There is no need for offering of suggestions,cervical dilation checks, or monitoring of progress in any way. If left to her own intuition and self-guidance, a comfortable and relaxed woman can birth her baby is a very short period of time.

A baby being born expects his mother to be able to relax and listen to the cues of her body so that he can make the passage as easily as possible.

Medical intervention is a self-fulfilling prophecy. Medical intervention prevents progression of the birth process, which in turn creates complications and safety issues, making complications likely and more serious medical intervention, such as C-section, "necessary." Well-nourished and relaxed mothers who give birth without hindrance from anyone, including medical professionals, are extremely unlikely to experience complications in labor.

Fear & Stress – Fear is the third of the four main causes of complications in pregnancy and childbirth. The body's natural response to fear and stress is extremely detrimental to the laboring mother. It can slow or shut down labor entirely, and has the capacity to cause pain and trauma as well.

*"Like all placental mammals, humans experience a slowing
down of contractions and delayed labor when they are
emotionally or cognitively stressed. The presence of multiple*

strangers in the delivery room is the norm for North American hospital births – the doctor, who may or may not be known to the woman, the labor nurses on duty, medical students, orderlies, and so on. If the woman is stressed by being surrounded by strangers, and not in control of her own body and actions, this may lead to delayed labor, which often leads to more interventions."

~Katherine A. Dettwyler

When survival and physical wellbeing are threatened, the body responds by shutting down all bodily systems apart from those deemed "necessary" for survival – this is called "fight or flight" or the "acute stress response." This response is very appropriate if, for instance, you were about to be eaten by a shark. It sends a rapid boost of energy into your body's musculature and increases the breath rate, blood pressure and blood sugar, while at the same time suppressing the immune system, the digestive system, the sexual organs (including the uterus,) and any other part of the body which does not serve the immediate purpose of defending or fleeing rapidly. This response is designed to save you in perilous or threatening situations. Birth, however, is not one of those situations.

This stress response creates enormous tension in the body, readying the body for quick and harsh action, which is completely adverse to the process of birth. Giving birth requires softness, relaxation, complete release of tension, and a totally calm and fear-free atmosphere. Birth is intense, but it is not tense. Fear takes away all of these necessary elements for pleasurable birth and replaces them with components which hinder the birth process, creating complications, pain, and trauma.

Stress and fear can have many causes. They can be caused by the mother feeling uneasy about certain people in her birthing space, not excluding people who she has invited into that space or who she has an intimate relationship with. Birthing is a sensitive process which, for the mother, can highlight subtle nuances that make the mother feel uncomfortable even if they would not otherwise. Stress can also be caused by the mother feeling uncomfortable or awkward about her birthing body, or about performing normal bodily functions like peeing or pooping in front of others. In order to avoid fear and stress in these situations, the mother needs to have a clear understanding with everyone who she has invited to her birth, that she is entitled to ask anyone to leave at any time, and that if asked, they are to leave quietly without any drama.

Other common causes of fear and stress include the threat of unwanted medical intervention, threats of moving the mother to another location or birthing space, or any practice which is occurring against the mothers expressed or unexpressed wishes, including others talking, watching her closely, touching her or not touching her, etc. In order to avoid fear and stress in these situations, it is up to the mother to communicate her wishes and intentions very clearly and directly, to anyone involved, both before the birth and as an unwanted situation is occurring or about to occur. It is up to all others involved in the birth to completely respect the mother's wishes and intentions, and not to question her authority in any situation.

Another common cause of stress and fear in childbirth is a mother's, (or anyone else's,) deep seated fear of the birth process itself. When a birthing mother is afraid of the birth process, sensing that it puts her or her coming baby in danger, she will be tense, on alert, and not able to relax her body or her emotions to let her baby pass through her. Fear of the birth process can cause many physical complications.

"I once worked with a couple who intellectually seemed to want to have a home birth, but who, on a lot of levels, seemed very afraid of birth. Despite my efforts to help them address their anxieties, they insisted that they were comfortable with birth and wanted to have the baby at home. When the woman finally went into labor, a couple of weeks past due, her blood pressure rose dramatically. We

chose to go to the hospital for the birth, where her blood
pressure normalized upon arrival. When I mentioned this
phenomenon to the attending nurse midwife... she confirmed
it, remarking that women can and do psychologically create
symptoms that land them in the hospital if that is where
they truly feel safer."

~Aviva Romm

Fear of the birth process itself is not conducive to an unassisted birth. Unhindered birthing requires a deep trust in the body and in the process of birth as safe. Fearful thoughts do not pose a problem, as long as you know that these thoughts do not hold any power over you. Fearful thoughts become a problem only when they are felt as stress in the emotions or the body. Thoughts do not affect your body, unless you let them. You can tell when your body is stressed – you can feel it in your muscles, your legs, and your stomach. If this feeling occurs when you think about the birth process, then you may be holding deep beliefs that birth is not safe. In order to avoid the possibility of a fearful labor, it is essential to acknowledge if you are holding any such beliefs and if so, to address them.

"Fear is always the result of an unquestioned past imagined
as a future."

~ Byron Katie

Women with a deep trust in the birth process are not likely to experience this bodily stress during the birthing process. Well-nourished women with a deep trust in their bodies to give birth will most likely experience the birth process as a blissful intensity.

Most often, fear-induced birth complications occur when the mother is experiencing fear. This is not always the case, however. *Anyone* experiencing fear, stress, or tension in the birthing space can affect the overall energy of the space, and in turn affect the mother and her birthing capabilities.

Ina May Gaskin, in her book "Spiritual Midwifery," recounts a story of a birth she attended where the mother's labor was stalled. The mother was experiencing regular contractions, but not making any progress. Ina May and the woman tried to work through a number of issues that may have been causing the tension, with no results. Finally, Ina May decided to try asking the husband to leave, as a last resort. The husband, who had been holding and supporting his wife from behind as she labored, left the room and decided to use the bathroom, since he had been holding in his need to pee for quite some time. As soon as he left, the woman was able to progress to full dilation and birthed her baby in a short time. Why? Ina May believed that the husband not urinating when he needed to caused him to feel tension in his body. Since he was not only in the space, but right up against the mother holding that tension, it carried over to the mother and affected her ability to give birth without her even realizing it. In order to avoid this, make sure everyone in the birthing space knows to attend to their needs and address their own fears.

Denial of Instincts – Being out of touch with or denying bodily instincts is the fourth reason that complications occur during childbirth. A birthing mother is usually very in tune with her body's needs, and listening to those needs often comes as second nature. In some cases, however, a mother may be accustomed to ignoring or denying her instincts due to social conditioning. Being out of touch with instincts or denying those instincts can inhibit the birth process. This can slow, stall, or stop labor entirely and could lead to complications.

Being out of touch with the body occurs through consistent denial of the body's needs. After years of denying your body proper nourishment, proper sleep, or proper elimination practices, you cease to be able to fully recognize when those needs arise. They become distant inklings rather than the clear sensations that they are meant to be. When you are out of touch with your body's needs on a daily basis, it may be difficult to hear that inner voice during labor – the voice that says "a warm bath is what I need" or "get me out of the bath!" or "get on your hands and knees!" Being able to hear that voice is so important during labor.

If you are out of touch with your body, you can begin to re-learn. Pay attention to your body's needs. Learn to recognize the moment you need to go pee – the moment you are thirsty – the moment you are ready to go to sleep. Learn to act on these bodily needs as soon as you are able, rather than putting these needs off until it is convenient.

Inhibition, or denial of instincts, occurs when a mother feels uncomfortable acting upon her instincts. This could occur for many reasons. For example, the mother could feel uncomfortable acting on certain impulses in front of others during labor. If this is the case, it is a good idea to ask those people who she feels uncomfortable around to leave. There is plenty of time in life for learning to cope with social inhibition; giving birth does not have to be one of those times.

A mother might also deny an instinct during labor if she thinks the instinct's call to action is silly or unnecessary. For example, during the birth process you might feel a need to be in a different room, a very strong need, but your rational mind may kick in and say, "that room is not prepared for me to birth in" or "there is no good reason for me to go there." Giving birth is not a rational process, and there is no need for rational thought to hinder or inhibit intuition. There may not be a clear reason why your body is telling you to do a certain thing, but it is important to listen to your intuition anyways. Trying to be 'rational' can be detrimental. As Ina May Gaskin says, a woman giving birth "becomes less of an individual personality and more like an elemental force, like a tornado, a volcano, an earthquake, or a hurricane, with its own laws of behavior…. You can't reason with an elemental force."

Another common reason for denying an impulse is inflexibility. One of the best birth stories that I read during my first pregnancy illustrates this point perfectly. In this story, the mother was planning a water birth. They had a midwife throughout the pregnancy, but planned not to call her when labor began – it was an intentional unassisted birth. When labor finally began, the woman asked her husband to fill the birthing pool. Once filled, she got into the pool and felt very relaxed and at ease. She stayed in the pool for a long time, and after a while noticed that she was feeling a bit more pain with each contraction. She had a feeling that it might be a good idea to get out of the pool, but ignored it because she thought her baby was close to being born, and she wanted him to have a water birth. The pain got worse and worse, until it was almost unbearable. She did not know what to do. She was desperate! Finally, she describes her body basically "throwing itself" out of the pool. Her body would no longer tolerate her inflexible mind denying the impulse to get out of the pool, and as she describes, her body acted of its own accord.

Many women have an idea of how birth is supposed to look; it is supposed to be a water birth, a lotus birth, or a "Frederick Leboyer" birth. The father is supposed to catch the baby, or the mother is supposed to catch the baby herself. There is nothing wrong with having these ideas about birth. The ideas can be quite nice. They only become a problem when they cause inflexibility. Inflexibility is rigidity. Birth is not rigid. It does not follow a plan. It does not conform. Birth has its own path – the baby, on her way into the world, has her own plans. It is important to be flexible during labor, and let labor follow its own course.

Without fear, medical intervention, the physical effects of poverty, or denial of instincts, birth is truly unhindered. Complications arise when the birth process is hindered, either circumstantially, by people attending the birth, or by the mother herself. When a woman giving birth is well-nourished, physically healthy, confident, totally relaxed, in-touch with her body, untouched by medical professionals except at her expressed desire, and respected by all present at her birth, then the birthing energy is allowed to flow freely and in all of its power. Unhindered birth energy is an extraordinarily beautiful thing.

Birth & Death

The idea of dying, or of someone we love dying, is often frightening. It is often perceived as unknown territory – unfamiliar – a loss of the consciousness that we experience in life. Death is the result that we often refer to when we say that something is unsafe. The safety of birth is defined by the maternal and infant mortality rate. The idea of maternal or infant death in childbirth is a huge component of many women's fear of giving birth.

All childbirth statistics point to the inherent safety of childbirth. For mothers, childbirth is just a bit safer than driving a car. For infants, the rate of death is higher, ranging from around 0.3% to around 4% in the United States. Maternal and infant death rates vary depending on the mother's health as well as where and with whom a woman chooses to give birth. The general trend points to the overwhelming majority of women and children living through the birth process, and yet, some women and some children do die.

Whether they choose a hospital birth, a midwife-attended homebirth, or an unassisted birth, some women and some infants will die in childbirth. There is so much controversy about the safety of homebirth vs. the safety of hospital birth. There are extremely strong and often hostile opinions coming from both sides of this debate. Although I have my own opinion, I personally do not want to have anything to do with this debate. I feel this debate is part of the issue, really – the issue being a widespread fear of death.

When it comes down to it, we must face the fact that we are all mortal. We will all die someday, and avoidance of this fact is what causes fear of death. Once you accept that death is inevitable at some point for each and every one of us, life becomes all the more vibrant in its temporality. Living life in fear of death is no way to live.

Just as the birth process has its own flow, so does the cycle of life. I know this to be true, and I don't let my fear or a cultural fear of death interfere with the path of my heart, which is to birth at home, with family, and in joy. I choose this way of birth because I believe it is the best choice for my family, and I truly believe that it is as safe as any.

Women who choose to birth without assistance are often told they are reckless for their choice. Why? No pregnant woman is told they are reckless for choosing to drive a car during pregnancy. Unless maybe if they are Amish.

~

A mother births her baby boy pre-maturely. She knows he will soon die, but out of love she chooses not to take the baby to the hospital. She chooses hold him, to soothe him, to love him with all of her being – to give the infant the gift of her pure, absolute, and unwavering tenderness and affection during those last moments of his life.

Some say that baby might have lived, and that the mother is therefore responsible for his death. My question to those people is, is extended life always better? Is the quality of a long life different from that of a short life? Is death so terrible that it must be prevented at all costs?

I say that a loving mother has every right to decide what is right for her newborn. That newborn is strongly connected to his mother. She will feel his pain. She will feel powerless and intense sadness.

In the case of the premature newborn boy who dies at home in his mother's arms, who is to say that those moments of life with his mother were not just as spacious and beautiful as the years of life he would have experienced if he had grown into an adult?

Our culture is so terrified of death that we often don't even stop to question these things. So let's question them! Why is it better to live 100 years than it is to live 10 minutes? Is there really any difference at all?

Although I feel strongly that there is nothing to fear in death, it does not mean that I do not feel incredible grief for mothers who have lost their babies, or babies who have lost their mothers, or families who have lost both.

I have read many stories of mothers who give birth to pre-mature babies, and slowly, over many weeks, watch their infants lose their life in the NICU. I have seen so many beautiful and heartbreaking pictures of premature babies in their mother's arms for the first time after weeks of failed attempts to keep them alive, just moments before they die.

I have also read stories of mothers who give birth prematurely and their baby, after weeks of watching and waiting, finally comes through alive. My own cousin, who I love very strongly, was one of those babies. She would not be here today to experience the beauty of life if it were not for her mother's choice.

I do not believe one mother's choice in these cases is better than another, as long as her choice is made in love. Still, the questions in my heart remain: Is extended life always better? How can those of us who have not died know? Why is it any more of a moral issue if a mother chooses to hold her baby in love as he dies, than it is if she takes him to the hospital in an attempt to save his life? I feel they are only choices – choices made by the mother, the woman whose connection to her infant is stronger than anyone's – if there is any right or wrong, it exists only for the mother, who knows in her heart what is right for her child.

When it's all said and done, is death really so unfamiliar? The "future" is unfamiliar, and yet we do not agonize about tomorrow – in fact, "tomorrow" is often an exciting prospect. In sleep, we often lose consciousness, and yet we do not agonize about going to sleep – in fact, it is often a welcome rest, a relaxation and surrender into unconsciousness. Life and death are not separate things. Life and death are part of one cyclical, beautiful, seamless whole.

~

"To see a World in a Grain of Sand,

and a Heaven in a Wild Flower,

Hold Infinity in the palm of your hand,

and Eternity in an hour."

~William Blake

Social Childbirth

Although the process of birth is essentially the same for all placental mammals, there is a sharp contrast in birthing practices between non-human mammalian species and humans. The difference lies in whether the mother chooses to birth her young in a social environment or to birth her young in solitude. Most mammals, even other primates, choose to seclude themselves from the social group when labor begins.

> *"A pregnant sheep, which is normally a herd dweller, will separate herself from the flock when birth becomes imminent. A rhesus monkey will move away from her group to the edge of the forest and choose a well-camouflaged hiding place in which to give birth. The rat, which is normally a nocturnal prowler, gives birth during the day to increase the chances that she'll be unobserved. And the horse, which is normally a daytime grazer, gives birth during the night for the same reason."*

> *~Chris Kresser*

It seems as though the inherent nature of an animal as social has nothing to do with whether she chooses to birth in a social environment. Sheep, apes, and monkeys, who are all very social animals, all choose to birth in solitude; why are humans different? Why do the overwhelming majority of women in today's culture choose to birth with other humans in her presence?

Human social birth does not necessarily mean hospital birth. Social birth means any birth which occurs in the presence of other humans, so that could include hospital birth, homebirth, or freebirth. The only type of solitary human birth is freebirth in which a woman separates herself from all other humans. Although there are some traditional cultures that very successfully preserved the practice of solitary birthing, most human cultures developed traditions of other women being present at births occurring in their tribe – these women were grown, usually older than the birthing mother – usually it was the birthing woman's own mother, her aunt, her grandmother, etc.

Many anthropologists argue that the onset of birth as a social event was due to the inherent dangers of human birth. In the 1980's, anthropologist Wenda Trevathan was the first to argue that social birthing became an evolutionary advantage when humans began to walk upright. Many others jumped on board this new theory. They said that birth became more complicated and dangerous with changes to the pelvis during this stage of human development. According to this theory, these pelvic changes required the infant to turn in the birth canal in order to successfully pass through it, and rather than facing the mother during birth, the baby faced toward the back of the mothers body. According to this theory, this made it difficult for the mother to catch and care for her seconds-old infant after birth, creating more possible complications and requiring birth to become a social act.

This theory, however, was conceived before recent intensive observation of the birth process of chimpanzees. Researchers in a 2011 Japan study developed very intimate relationships with captive chimpanzees, sleeping and living with them, in the hopes of being witness to a chimpanzee birth. Before this study, no-one had ever witnessed a live chimpanzee birth, as chimpanzees prefer to birth in solitude, without observation. These researchers were eventually able to witness three live births. They found that in three out of three births, the baby was born facing away from the mother. Dr. Satoshi Hirata, one of the researchers involved in the study, said after the study that "anthropologists have argued that the fact that human babies are born facing away from the mothers has led to 'midwifery'. Our observation tells us that this is not true. We tend to think that we are unique, without knowing about other animals."

So, if humans did not develop social birthing practices due to our change to bipedalism , then why? Why did the traditional cultures across the globe develop social birthing practices, when chimpanzees did not?

No one will ever truly know, but I strongly believe that social childbirth developed, not because of any inherent danger in the birth process, but because of the evolution of human capacity to experience life events as spiritual rites of passage. A woman's first experience of childbirth marks a monumental change in her life, just as does her first menstrual period, or the onset of menopause. Pagan traditions often reference the three stages of womanhood: maiden, mother, and crone. A child becomes a 'maiden' when she enters sexual maturity, a mother when she bears a child, and a crone when sexual maturity finally wanes. These are all very important changes in a woman's life, and I believe that the development of social childbirth traditions is due to a developmental shift in humans such that they desired to celebrate the sacred and monumental events of life. This change in human history marked the beginning of intentional burial, of sacred ceremony, and of "rites of passage," – moments in a man or woman's life where he or she was initiated into an older, more mature and more spiritually conscious class of their gender. This is why traditionally, childbirth attendants were always female and had always experienced childbirth for themselves. Childbirth is a rite of passage.

Of course, women attending a birth can also help the laboring mother if she desires, and this may have actually proven advantageous and developed into a practice of its own, but in my opinion this is not why social childbirth developed to begin with. In my opinion, mothers attended childbirth to celebrate the sacredness of the event, and to initiate the birthing woman into motherhood.

Male Birth Attendants

In traditional cultures, men were not involved in the birth process at all. In many cases the father did not even see his child until a week or so after the birth. This ancient tradition contrasts sharply with most modern births, in which the father and other men are not only present as observers, but often play an important role in the birth process itself.

In Katherine Dettwyler's book "Cultural Anthropology & Human Experience," she cites an occasion in which a group of female Sudanese refugees from the Nuer tribe, some of whom were pregnant or already mothers, were shown a video depicting an average North American hospital birth. The Nuer women were shocked into laughter and screams to see the woman's husband by her side at the birth, and even more upset to see the man kiss and touch his wife during labor. One pregnant woman could not continue to watch the video, and ran from the room.

When once childbirth was fundamentally and interminably an event for women and women alone, it is now become an event for both sexes, and often seen as an opportunity for spiritual growth, vulnerability, and increased connectivity in the relationship of the mother and father.

Why the shift, and what does it mean? Are male birth attendants antithetical to birth itself, and should they be excluded? I don't believe so. This shift occurred due to the human shift from the tribal unit to the "family unit." Women, in most cases in modern cultures, no longer live with their mothers, sisters, grandmothers and aunts. The tribal unit has been dispersed – upon entering adulthood most humans leave their parents' homes in search of their own nuclear family unit. This unit often consists of a man, a woman, and their children. The adults in this unit develop an incredibly intimate bond out of necessity – they are the only adults present in their day-to-day home lives.

In traditional cultures, women had the chance to develop intensely intimate relationships with the women around them – their maternal elders or older sisters – and this made birth with these women easy. Today, there is often a disconnect between generations. Many, (although certainly not all,) women in today's culture would feel very uncomfortable giving birth in front of their mother, their sister, their aunt, or their grandmother, and so they turn to the only person whom they have developed that deeply intimate relationship with, their husband or partner, to be their companion during labor.

I do not believe there is anything wrong with men attending childbirth, unless the men see themselves as 'in charge' or are in any way domineering. As long as a man knows that the birthing mother is the complete authority, then I see this development as just an interesting occurrence in human social evolution.

Personally, I long for that tribal setting – an interwoven clan, a network of human cooperation and love – but as that is not the case for me or for many other modern women, then birthing with those who we do feel truly intimate with, no matter what their gender or familial relation, seems like a workable option with its own unique beauties and advantages.

Modern Solitary Childbirth

S ocial birthing may have become a tradition in many cultures, but there are still some cultures where it never took hold. Until very recently in the course of human history, women in these cultures chose to seclude themselves during labor and childbirth. Accounts of these traditional 'solo' births describe pain-free and easy labors, affirming the notion that social childbirth did not develop out of necessity due to the complications of human birth, but for other, perhaps spiritual reasons.

Traditionally in some First Nations tribes of Canada, where women often chose to birth with no assistance, preparations would be made beforehand to ensure the woman had a safe and warm place to go during labor. This took the form of a birthing hut or space, fashioned in the woods a month or two before the expected onset of labor. Often in these cases, the woman would prepare this space herself. When the first signs of labor began, she would isolate herself in this space, where all preparations for the birth had been made beforehand.

The !Kung of Africa had similar traditions.

In modern culture, it is rare for a woman to choose to birth without any assistance, but not as rare as you might think. Women who choose solitary freebirth do so for belief-based reasons, for heart-felt reasons, or for circumstantial reasons, (i.e. an unstable relationship.) Sometimes, like in the case of my son's birth, a 'solo' freebirth happens accidentally. I planned to give birth with my partner, Joey, present, but he was asleep at the time, and the labor happened very fast.

For me, birthing in solitude left me completely uninhibited and able to act directly, without second thought or reserve, on all of my instincts and impulses. It was such a primal experience, and taught me of the power of truly unhindered birth. Although some say that solo unassisted birth is reckless, I do not believe it is so. Many of our ancestors chose to do this, and if you feel called to this too, then there may be a very good reason; many women find that birthing in the presence of others, even lovers or close friends, can be inhibiting in some way.

Birthing in solitude does not mean that total isolation is necessary – it does not mean that you need to follow some idea or belief to an extreme. It may just mean sectioning off a room or a few rooms in your house and asking others not to disturb you unless you ask in some way for assistance, or it may mean having a friend on call to come and help you if you decide you want help. When I gave birth to Micah without assistance, I had a signal worked out with a friend who I was living with at the time; I would turn the lights on if I needed any help. She was putting her baby to sleep in a cabin just outside of the house that I gave birth to Micah in. After Micah was born, I suddenly felt very cold and I wanted help. I turned on a light, and she came, along with my partner, Joey. Together, they built a fire in the woodstove, cut the umbilical cord when I was ready, made me a bowl of cereal, and prepared a temporary bed for Micah and I to sleep in that night so that we didn't have to walk outside in the cold (to the cabin where I normally slept.)

A part of me wishes I had waited just a few minutes to turn on the light – waited just a bit longer to bond with Micah in the darkness before asking for assistance. I am, however, so grateful for their help. It would have been different in that immediate post-partum period had I been totally alone, but I know of women who have done it, and who have been grateful for their experiences as well.

Listen, Trust, & Choose

O ut of all this, I have gleaned one thing: trust your intuition. Throughout human history, where and with whom a woman chooses to give birth has gone through enormous transformations – from solitude, to social, to midwife-attended woman-centered births, to hospital births, to modern family homebirths, and everywhere in-between.

The process of birth is versatile in that it can occur in many types of physical and social (or un-social) settings – the only factors that are required for a successful birth are a well-nourished & healthy mother, a setting in which the mother feels safe and relaxed, and the ability of the mother to birth without hindrance from others or from her own mind. *Only the mother will know how to create such a space for herself.*

A mother's deep knowing will make clear to her what needs to fall into place for her birth. She will prepare herself in her own way. When labor begins, she will know who should be there, who should not, and where exactly it will feel most comfortable to give birth.

Birth is as different for each woman as each woman is different.It is a personal process, one that is deeply ingrained in our body's memory. Listen to your body, to your feelings. Trust these feelings. Make your birth choices according to your own wisdom, and you will choose what is best for you and your child.

PART IV:

Childbirth

& Postpartum

"Endless moons, an opaque universe, thunder, tornadoes,
the quaking earth…. life was there, a transparent pearl, a
star revolving slowly on its own axis."

~ Shan Sa

The end of pregnancy is a new beginning – the birth of your child – the passage into motherhood. Giving birth, the channel between pregnancy and motherhood, is the most intense, beautiful, vulnerable and ecstatic moment of a woman's life, apart, perhaps, from her own birth. This dance of mother and infant is an elemental happening – a profound happening – a force beyond control or reason. There is no other moment as opening as childbirth – your body opens, your mind opens, your heart opens – wider than ever before – it is a true communion with the divine, a temporary glimpse into the true, unadulterated, unreserved power of life.

The Process of Childbirth

"Fear? Oh, no! You feel you're protected as if standing in a magic circle where nothing can touch you. You are under the protection, the blessings of infinite Light and Love embodied in your child. Yes, you are under the protection of this little one on its way to you."

~ "Letter from an Older Woman, Canada," from Frederick Leboyer's "Art of Giving Birth."

Onset of Labor & the "First Stage"

"All natural birth has a purpose and a plan; who would think of tearing open the chrysalis as the butterfly is emerging? Who would break the shell to pull the chick out?"

~ Marie Mongan

The Onset: A few weeks before the onset of labor, the baby "drops," meaning that she descends deeper into your pelvis in preparation for birth. This results in increased pressure on the lower belly & bladder and decreased pressure on the stomach and lungs. Many mothers notice that their vagina is more lubricated during these last three weeks, and some may even experience preparatory contractions or false labor. During this period, you may feel a deep sense of wanting your home to be complete & ready for the birth. You might find yourself falling asleep each night awaiting the beginnings of labor, or, you might not think about it much at all. If this isn't your first pregnancy, your baby may never drop noticeably.

The onset of labor comes in many ways. For most, the energy of birth is a steady rise, a slow tide coming in, almost imperceptible at first. It rises until it is undeniably flowing through your whole being, consuming & alive. Once it is recognized, the slow and steady rising often quickly becomes more rapid and powerful.

For others, labor starts suddenly – the breaking of waters, a gushing of fluid, and labor is at once strong, steady, and continual.

For some, it comes and goes – the gentle lapping of waves over days or weeks, touching, but never really entering the body. It is there and then it is not; a gentle ebb and flow, until it finally and truly enters, and the energy continues to flow more and more rapidly.

Signals of the beginning of labor vary from person to person. Breaking of waters is usually a very good indicator that labor will soon begin. The amniotic fluid (waters) is sometimes clear, and sometimes green or brown. Green or brown fluid means that the baby has had a bowel movement in-utero, and some say that this is a sign of fetal distress. Gloria Lemay and many others, however, disagree, saying that a bowel movement in-utero is actually *almost never* a sign of fetal distress.

If labor does not begin within an hour of your waters breaking, this is called "premature rupture of membranes," (orPROM.) Most women with PROM go into labor within 24 hours. Avoid vaginal exams, sex, or any other practice which may encourage bacteria, since the breaking of waters without going into labor can increase the risk of an infection. One of the best things you can do to ensure a strong bag of waters is to eat a diet very rich in Vitamin C throughout pregnancy. Strawberries, most other berries, kale, oranges, rose hips, tomatoes, bell peppers, cilantro – these are just a few foods and herbs that are naturally high in vitamin C. This ensures a thick amniotic sac and a thick umbilical cord, which are both beneficial during the birth process. Ruptured membranes, in many cases, can heal themselves. Herbs which I'll discuss in the coming chapters can assist with this.

For others, the "mucus plug" becomes dislodged and this signifies the onset of labor. The mucus plug is somewhat gelatinous and mucus-like, clear, translucent white, or cream colored, sometimes tinged with a bit of blood. Losing your mucus plug does not mean that you'll go into labor, and if you lose it early it can re-form, but for many this signifies the onset of the birth process.

For others, almost imperceptible contractions signify the beginning of labor – these may feel like menstrual cramps, minor back aches, or an urge to have a bowel movement or sit on the toilet. For women whose labor is signified by contractions, the mucus plug may never clearly be seen during labor, and the waters can break at any time. Sometimes, like in the case of my daughter, the amniotic sac does not break until just before crowning or even after birth.

Each of my three labors began with contractions, but with my firstI did not realizefor a long time what they were – I just felt intermittent cramps and urges to use the bathroom until I realized it was labor, and upon realizing, the energy seemed to amplify greatly. Peacy's waters never broke, and I chose to break them when she was crowning. Micah was born falling from his amniotic sac – his waters never broke either. With my third birth, I finally had the pleasure of knowing what it felt like for my waters to break during labor – incredible!

Once labor begins: Essentially, giving birth happens of its own accord, but it is helpful to appreciate what is necessary and expected of you in the process. It is helpful to understand that nothing needs to be done, but rather, if you let go of doing, you will experience your body acting by itself.

> *"There is power that comes to women when they give birth.*
> *They don't ask for it, it simply invades them. Accumulates*
> *like clouds on the horizon and passes through, carrying the*
> *child with it."*

> *~ Sheryl Feldman*

The energy of birth can be described in so many ways. What are most commonly referred to as "contractions" have many more names that I feel are much more appropriate. I like the terms 'rush,' 'peak,' and 'wave' because they refer to the energy of a contraction rather than the physical muscular action of the uterus, but for the sake of clarity, I will call them contractions.

If timed, contractions are usually spaced evenly and become closer and closer together. (Timing of contractions is not in any way necessary, and can be a hindrance if it is distracting to the mother.)

The sensation of a contraction is difficult to describe – there is something exciting in it, opening, loosening – deep and grounding, like a force pulling you deep into the earth or deep into yourself. There is also a very powerful energy which, as some might say, you learn to ride like a wave. As labor progresses, the waves get bigger, stronger, and more powerful, and riding them becomes increasingly intense.

Some describe the sensations of contractions as menstrual cramp-like; others describe them as uncomfortable backaches, gas pain-like, or similar to an urge to have a bowel movement. The sensation of a contraction is similar to these things in some ways, but using these analogies to describe contractions is misleading – it is like trying to describe the sensation of an orgasm to someone who has never experienced an orgasm. (I remember a friend telling me as a young woman who had not yet reached orgasm during sex, that an orgasm felt like a sneeze.) A contraction is a contraction – it feels like a contraction, just like an orgasm is an orgasm, and feels like an orgasm.

During labor, the cervix softens, thins, and gradually, with each contraction, it opens. This opening is greatly facilitated by the relaxation of the mother through her contractions. In order to open fully, a mother should not fight the contractions or resist them, but embrace them. Embrace them fully with no opposition, and surrender to the power that they hold. Contractions do not require that you do anything – they require that you let go of doing, let go of any attempt to control your body, and truly surrender to the awesome power of childbirth.

The period from the onset of labor until the cervix is fully dilated is called the "first stage" of labor. Some women experience very quick first stages, and some slow. An average modern 'first stage' for a first time mother lasts from 4 to 24 hours. This is divided into "early labor" which is mild and in some cases can even continue for 2 or 3 days, and "active labor" which is more intense. By itself, active labor does not usually last more than 8 hours, but in some cases it can.

Your concept of time becomes very distorted during labor, and many hours can seem like no time at all. Since we lived without electricity during the birth of my first child, we did not have a clock to check the time. I am very grateful for this. In my subsequent births, even though we lived with clocks in the house, I didn't think to look at them.

Many women say that first births last longer than subsequent births, as was my case, but this is not always the case by any means. Each birth has its own unique time frame and energy.

> *"Attending births is like growing roses. You have to marvel at the ones that just open up and bloom at the first kiss of the sun but you wouldn't dream of pulling open the petals of the tightly closed buds and forcing them to blossom to your time line."*
>
> ~ *Gloria Lemay*

Why do some births take longer than others? For as many reasons as there are births – each birth is completely unique. There are some overlapping factors, though – some births are just slow. They start out calmly, rise steadily, and just last a long time for no other reason than that the baby is taking his or her time.

Some long labors, though, are caused by a physical, mental or emotional barrier. Distinguishing between physical, mental, and emotional is in many ways deceptive – these "parts" are not really parts, but different ways of looking at the whole of your being. The distinction is only in the different perspective, which can be helpful if you are trying to work through a barrier. As Ina May Gaskin says, "since body and mind are one, sometimes you can fix the mind by working on the body, and sometimes you can fix the body by working on the mind."

Some examples of barriers to a quick labor include social inhibition, bodily tension, fear of the intensity of opening, fear of vulnerability, and fear or tension in general from the mother or from others in the birthing space. If the mother is unsure about become a mother, or has conflicting feelings about the father of her child, these feelings can also stall a labor until they are expressed.

Occasionally, the position of the baby can slow labor. I'll discuss this briefly in the coming chapters.

In hospitals, it has become commonplace to restrict food and drink during labor. This is not because it is helpful for the mother or because it is in some way harmful to eat and drink during labor –it is hospital policy because, in the case that the mother is "put under," it would be detrimental for her to vomit.

Consuming food and drinking fluids during labor, as the needs arise, is imperative. Women who experience short & intense labors may never feel the need to eat or drink, but during longer labors it is very important to maintain electrolyte balance by drinking fluids and eating when hungry. This ensures optimal muscle functioning and energy levels for the birthing mother.

As active labor progresses, it becomes more and more intense, more and more powerful, until the cervix is fully dilated. The segment at the end of the first phase of labor, as the body is approaching full openness and your baby is readying himself to pass into your birth canal, is called "transition."

Transition and the Myth of 10cm: When contractions begin to get very intense nearing full cervical dilation, some women experience them as overpowering or too intense. Know, in these times, that they will not overpower you – they will rock you, shake you, and move you, but in the end they are a part of you. The power of the contractions, as amazing as it may seem, comes from you! Do not be afraid of that power – be in awe of it; marvel at this incredible force which you never knew you had!

> *"Nearly every mother, at some point in her labor, feels that it is going to be impossible to give birth. If [you know] that this thought is likely to occur, [you] can take it less seriously when it comes."*
>
> *~Ina May Gaskin*

For many women, this thought occurs during transition. Transition is incredibly powerful, like an earthquake or a huge wave churning through your body. It does not usually last very long, maybe only a few minutes or even seconds, but that power is so absolute that it is extraordinarily memorable. Transition marks the separation between the first and the second stages of labor.

We often hear that full cervical dilation is equal to 10cm. When we look a little more closely at this, it becomes obvious that it is not true – it is only a way of talking about full dilation. Some women never reach 10cm, and some women dilate well beyond 10cm. Every woman's body is unique, every pregnancy is unique, every baby is unique, and every birth is unique.

Vaginal exams during birth have become commonplace. These exams aim to identify the progress of the labor – how close a woman is to the second phase. In my opinion, these exams don't have a lot to tell, and if performed by another, can actually hinder the birth process.

Cervical dilation can change rapidly. Labor can progress very unevenly. Perhaps the first few centimeters of cervix take many hours to dilate, while the last few only take a few minutes. Or, perhaps the first few centimeters take minutes, while the rest take many hours. Cervical checks can bring a false sense of 'progress' (or lack thereof) to the mother. Birth, by all means, does not follow a formula!! Trust in the process – trust that your body has its own formula.

The "Second Phase" & the Birth

"I would consider moments of my birth experience to be orgasmic, but not in the typical sense, more like heart orgasms, like when I felt my son enter my birth canal right before crowning, that was a total heart orgasm, the coolest thing ever. We need more definitions for these kinds of things I think!"

~ Leah Fisher

The second phase of labor begins after full dilation, when your baby enters your birth canal. This phase can be very quick, lasting only a few minutes, or it can last up to a few hours. This phase is ecstatic – your baby is so close! You can feel her like never before, descending, coming closer and closer to her birth. When she finally parts the lips of your vagina and you reach down to touch her, there is no moment that compares to this! And yet, the entirety of this stage of labor is like that – indescribable infinite bliss. I remember gasping in pure joy through this phase – never in my life have I been so open – so inexplicably close to the light and love of heaven.

This phase is often referred to as the "pushing" phase. The uterine muscles contract to help push the baby down through the birth canal. During this phase, your body knows just what to do, and voluntarily pushing without feeling a very strong impulse to push is not necessary for most women.

It is a common myth that very hard and arduous effort is required of the mother during this phase – TV shows often depict sweaty, struggling moms pushing with all their might. However, in most unhindered births, the muscles of our bodies will automatically contract to push our babies out. For most women, this phase works best if it is left alone – left to be effortless – left to the intelligence of the body. However, some women say that their bodies never pushed involuntarily, and that a conscious effort was required.

As the baby begins to crown, your body will tell you what position to assume. For me, 'hands-and-knees' was always my favorite throughout the second stage.

Crowning is such a passionate moment. Your baby is bridging the gap between her world, the soft muffled wet world inside of you, the only space she has ever known, and the world outside. You are about to meet her – to hold her for the first time, to comfort her through this monumental transition, and to experience an enormous transition yourself – the transition into motherhood! This moment is beyond words.

For some women, especially women who have already given birth or who tend to birth small babies, the baby comes very, very quickly. If a baby is born too quickly, this can sometimes result in a perennial tear. It is hard to fathom holding back during this phase – it is such an exhilarating moment and you are, after all, about to see your baby for the first time! Tears heal. Although they are uncomfortable, there are worse things in life, so if you can't contain your excitement and the baby comes very quickly, then do not worry. Some midwives advise, however, to let the baby crown and be birthed a bit more slowly. If you want to avoid tearing, it may be a good idea to let yourself stretch once or twice before your baby crowns, and for you or someone else present to support your perineum and gently hold the baby's head as he comes through, so that he doesn't come through all in one burst.

"It is really important at the time of crowning that the mother keeps both her throat and her mouth loose and relaxed. If the mother wants to know what she can do with her mouth to keep it loose, she can laugh or sing or say "I love you."

~ Ina May Gaskin

If your waters have not yet broken, then your baby will still be in the 'caul,' or amniotic sac. This means you have a strong sac, and it is actually beneficial for your baby – an intact caul prevents prolapse of the umbilical cord, and protects the baby until the very end of labor. My daughter began to crown with her sac still intact, but kept withdrawing back into the birth canal. It was not until we gently broke the membrane of the sac that she fully crowned and passed through me. Your intuition will tell you what is best – for me, breaking the sac at the very end of labor seemed to help immensely, and seemed to free her so that she could pass through more easily.

Once your baby's head is born, her body rotates by 90 degrees to the left or right. After this rotation, the shoulders and body may pass all at once, which is often the case with smaller babies, or the shoulders may take a few minutes to be born. If the latter is the case, the shoulders are usually born one at a time.

If the baby's shoulders become stuck anywhere along the way in the pelvis, this is called "shoulder dystocia." Shoulder dystocia most often occurs when the mother is lying on her back, but it can occur in other situations as well. The best thing you can do to relieve a stuck shoulder is to follow the instinctual movements of your body. Most of the time, movement is the key. The "gaskin maneuver" is also very popularamong midwives, for good reason, and simply involves immediately assuming the "hands-and-knees" position, which widens the pelvis. A variation on the Gaskin Maneuver is called the "running start": In the hands & knees position, you can bring one leg forward (as if bracing for the start of a marathon,) and rock your pelvis, or do whatever your body tells you to do in this position, and then switch legs. Learn more about this (or the "FlipFlop" technique,) on the "spinning babies" website, which is an amazing resource. If this alone does not help, you or someone with you can apply "gentle traction," as Ina May says, to the baby's posterior armpit if you can locate it. If this does not help, Ina May suggests that in extremely rare cases you may need to free the posterior arm before the baby can slide out. Shoulder dystocia is very rare in unhindered births.

When your baby's shoulders are born, the rest of him will slide out easily. You or someone else can catch him, or you can arrange a pile of soft towels for him to land on. In some cultures, women traditionally birthed alone by standing or squatting over a little low hammock, arranged beforehand, and letting the baby fall into it.

Many say that it is imperative to hold your baby to your chest immediately after birth. My feeling differs, slightly. I feel it is imperative to follow your intuition just after birth. If you intuitively reach out to hold your baby, then that is what is necessary. Some women, however, find that a short pause, an unhurried moment to calmly study and meet their newborn, is more important to them than immediate skin-to-skin.

Most newborns will breathe spontaneously. Suctioning is not usually necessary, and can be harmful if done without need.Newborns may breathe calmly and quietly, or they may breathe and cry. If they are not pink at birth, then they should begin to turn pink within the first minute.

If your baby does not breathe soon after birth, check for any mucus blocking the baby's nose and mouth, and check to make sure the umbilical cord is not around his neck. *If* there is mucus blocking his airway, you can gently suction it from his air passages with your mouth, and if the cord is around his neck, unwrap it as calmly as you can. Don't panic if your baby is not breathing just after birth – as long as you do not cut the umbilical cord prematurely, your baby is still receiving oxygenated blood from the placenta.

"A normal healthy baby should breathe within a half-minute to a minute after birth."

~Ina May Gaskin

Some babies just need a little stimulation to breathe. Hold her close to your skin, massage her, and make sure she is very warm. If you run your fingers over the souls of her feet, this can initiate a breathing reflex. If the baby is blue, white, limp, or seems lifeless, this may be a sign of severe asphyxia. Tell her you love her – speak to her

– tell her you want her to stay with you. Massage her and keep her warm. If you know her name, then say her name out loud. If your infant is still not breathing, you can use infant Cardio-pulmonary Resuscitation, (CPR,) or Neonatal Resurrection, (NRP,) techniques, which can both be learned in a class. If you feel there is hope and your baby is asking for life, then don't give up. If your intuition clearly tells you that your baby will not come back or that he is asking to be left in peace, then honor his wishes. In Spiritual Midwifery, Ina May Gaskin says that "cardio-pulmonary resuscitation continued for as long as 30 to 45 minutes has saved babies, without brain damage."

This section has conveyed quite a lot of 'information' about the second stage of birth. It might seem overwhelming. Don't try to memorize it, unless you want to. I share it only because some women want to feel prepared for birth by knowing what to do if certain unusual situations arise.

Those Infinite Moments just after Birth

Those moments just after birth are so magical. Your baby is so new – seeing this world for the first time, feeling air on his skin for the first time. There is nothing as deep as the eyes of a newborn, or as soft and perfect as his tiny body. For your baby to have the smoothest and most gentle transition possible, and to avoid shock and trauma, do all you can to mirror your internal environment – the environment of your womb.

A gentle transition into this new world can have a very beneficial impact on your newborn. The impact can last through those moments after birth, throughout his infancy, and some say even into adulthood. These moments build your infant's initial impressions of his new world – they shape his formative feelings about safety, comfort, and affection.

For the last nine months, your baby has grown to know your womb as his world. He has clearly heard the sound of your voice, and the muffled voices and sounds of your daily life. He has heard the beating of your heart, felt your body's warmth, and seen only dim light, made pink through the filter of your body. Mirroring this environment is the most loving thing you can do to ease this immense transition. Warmth, skin-to-skin, dim lighting or no lighting, and the soft, soothing sound of your voice all help to mirror this environment.

The room after birth should be as warm as possible, without being hot. You should be comfortable to be naked, and you should not feel cold. If you feel cold, your infant probably feels cold as well. He can be wrapped in blankets after birth, but you and your baby can also be wrapped together, which more closely resembles the environment he is used to – your womb.

Skin-to-skin contact is so important after birth. It provides continuity and a feeling of safety. It lets the infant know that you, his world, are still with him in this foreign environment.

The Umbilical Cord

During pregnancy, the umbilical cord is your baby's connection to you. It is a conduit – a channel which links you to your growing baby and sustains him. Through this channel, vitally potent blood passes from the placenta to your baby; this blood is oxygenated, and rich in nutrients. When the blood has been used, it passes back through the cord to the placenta, depleted of its vitality. This is how your baby breathes, eats, and takes in fluid while in-utero – the placenta supplies oxygen, fluids, and nutrients from the mother's bloodstream to the baby's bloodstream through the umbilical cord.

During the birth process, an unobstructed umbilical cord is essential to your baby's wellbeing after birth. Prolapse of the umbilical cord, although extremely rare, can occur. If this occurs, pressure from the baby's presenting part on the cord can cause the flow of oxygen to the baby to be restricted or cut off entirely. If this occurs, the baby needs to be born quickly to avoid brain damage or death. This occurs in an estimated 14 in 10,000 births, and will usually only occur when the amniotic sac ruptures prematurely. To ensure a strong amniotic sac, eat a nutrient-dense diet rich in vitamin C throughout pregnancy. Vitamin C will also ensure a thick, healthy umbilical cord.

Immediately after birth, your baby is still connected to you through the umbilical cord. Before the placenta detaches, blood, nutrients and oxygen are still passing through the cord from you to your baby. The cord can still be felt pulsating after birth, which usually signifies that a steady flow of blood is making its way to your baby. If your baby is otherwise not showing signs of life, but the cord is pulsing, this is a very good sign that he can be revived with massage, voice, warmth, and a little stimulation.

How to cut the cord: How to cut the cord depends on when you plan to cut it. If you plan to cut the cord within the first few hours after birth, or before it has gone totally limp, then you will need to clamp or tie the cord. The gentlest thing to use in this case is soft, 100% natural string. It can be hemp, cotton, linen, or some other natural material. Try not to use polyester string or metal or plastic clamps on a newborn's umbilical cord. Tying the umbilical cord, (tightly,) cuts off the flow of blood passing back and forth from your baby to the placenta, and ensures that once it is cut, the baby will not bleed out through the cord.

Once the cord has been tied or clamped, you can use something sharp to cut it. For example, you could use a knife or a sharp shell or a pair of scissors. You can sterilize a knife or scissors before cutting, if you wish, by holding the blade over a flame for a few seconds, until it becomes hot. Let it cool again before using it. One of the first natural birth stories I ever heard, told to me by my partner Joey, involved the umbilical cord being severed by the father's teeth. The story, which I found quite romantic, exciting, and beautiful, depicted a woman giving birth in the woods. When she was ready, her partner used his teeth to sever the cord. This is what other mammals do.

If and when to cut the cord: The connection through the umbilical cord after birth gives your baby a window of opportunity to transition from receiving oxygen through the cord to receiving it through his own brand new lungs. For this reason, cutting the cord immediately after birth has been shown to have very detrimental effects on the long-term health of the baby.

When cutting of the umbilical cord is delayed, this decreases the chance of iron-deficiency and anemia in the baby, and also ensures healthy circulation and red blood cell volume. In hospitals, many say that early clamping and cutting of the cord is necessary to ensure that the infant does not become jaundiced. Most in the homebirth world say that the cord should remain intact until it stops pulsing, as this is a clear physical sign that the baby has received what was necessary from the cord. Many women choose to wait a few hours before cutting the cord, until well after the birth of the placenta – they wait until the cord has turned white, gone totally limp, and become dry. In these cases, the cord is no longer transferring anything from the placenta to the baby, and does not even need to be tied. Others in recent years have begun a practice called "lotus birth," where the cord remains attached to the placenta and is carried with the baby until it falls off naturally. Proponents of lotus birth say that this is the gentlest transition possible for an infant coming earthside.

In my opinion, delayed cord cutting is an essential aspect of a smooth transition for your infant from womb to world. It gives him a chance to get used to his new lungs before severing his known oxygen supply. Early cutting forces his lungs to immediately carry the load for his whole body's oxygen requirements. Delayed cutting lets him receive essential blood, nutrients, and minerals from the placenta, which can help immensely in his first few months of life.

There is also an aspect to delayed cord cutting that is hard to put my finger on. Waiting to cut the cord seems like an act of respect for the mother-child bond – a token of the continuation of life from mother to child. While the placenta is still inside of the mother, the cord still unites her to her baby. Early severance seems abrupt – like an unexpected severance of that lingering unification of mother and child.

When it comes to cutting the cord, I use my intuition. In my three births, we waited to cut our children's umbilical cords until it felt right.

Traditionally, humans have many differing practices when it comes to cutting the cord, but as far as I know there are no traditional cultures that practice what is today known as "lotus birth." Both Susun Weed and Ina May Gaskin warn that if an umbilical cord stays attached for too long, or if it is "milked" after birth, that this can cause jaundice in your newborn.

There are so many differing opinions around this subject. My feeling is that the mother will intuitively know what is right for her newborn – she will feel in herself whether the cord should be cut in the first few minutes after birth, or the first few hours, or not at all. Whatever she chooses, I believe she has chosen perfectly for her child.

The "Third Phase," the Placenta, & Uterine Involution

The third phase of the birth process refers to the time from the moments after birth until the placenta is delivered. It is a common misconception that the birth process stops with the birth of a child. The uterus is still working after the baby is born, and will continue to contract until the entire birth process is complete. This third phase usually lasts only around five minutes, but it can last longer. As contractions continue after birth, they begin to reduce the size of the uterus. The placenta remains the same size while the uterine walls shrink, and the wall of the placenta which is attached to the uterine wall will eventually buckle and detach. A small quantity of deep red blood will typically come through the vagina as the placenta separates, and the placenta is usually born shortly thereafter.

Once the placenta has detached, more uterine contractions will push it through the cervix. The mother will have a full feeling in her birth canal, and can pass the placenta by standing or squatting over a basin.

The same relaxation required for labor and birth is necessary for the delivery of the placenta. The environment should be fear-free, comfortable, and soft so the uterus will continue to contract efficiently. Fear, intolerance or anxiety can all hinder this phase as much as they can during any other part of labor.

Usually the placenta is birthed within 10 minutes. For some, however, it takes longer. The time frame varies depending on who you ask – some sources say that the time frame for placental delivery is 30 to 45 minutes. Others say that as long as the mother is not bleeding heavily, the time frame extends to up to an hour. Some women report that their placentas took much longer to be birthed, even up to 6 hours, without any problems at all.

There are some non-invasive techniques, listed below, that can help encourage placental delivery.

Massaging the belly around the uterus can stimulate contractions and be greatly effective in expelling the placenta. If your baby will latch on, breastfeeding can also help – it stimulates oxytocin and promotes contractions. If your infant does not want to nurse, you can stimulate your nipples yourself or have someone else do it. You can also try standing, walking and letting gravity do the trick. Walking can help to stimulate contractions, and a standing position can help facilitate placental detachment. Squatting when a contraction comes can also be helpful.

If none of these methods work and you feel the need to act in some way, you can try and find other ways to stimulate abdominal contraction. You can induce sneezing or coughing, blow using your abdominal muscles, or if those do not work, you can try stimulating your gag reflex.

I want to stress, however, that unless something feels "off" or wrong, that there is absolutely no need to do anything about the placenta – your body will take care of it, if left unhindered.

According to Veronika Robinson, many traditional cultures used heat to expel the placenta. This reinforces the importance of warmth for both the mother and the child after the birth. "Some cultures, such as that of the Moroccans, traditionally use heat. They soak the severed end of the cord in oil that has been heated. The placenta falls out within a few minutes. Heat is also used by the Mexicans, who place a hot tortilla on the mother's side. The Cahuilla and Benua-Jakun encourage the mother to stand over a fire."

"Probably one of the most revealing and beautiful aspects of tribal cultures is that of patience. In all but the rarest of circumstances, they know that by being patient, all births will end well."

~Veronika Sophia Robinson

If something feels "off" and the placenta continues to adhere after attempting all of these methods, and if there is heavy bleeding, this could result in hemorrhage. There are herbal remedies which can be used in these cases, which I will discuss in section 4.7, "Herbs for Childbirth."

After placental birth the uterus will continue to contract for a few days. For first time mothers, the cramps that accompany these contractions are not usually painful. For some mothers, the pain of the contractions becomes worse with each successive child; this is because the muscles of the uterus can lose tone over time. Contractions after birth are also called "afterpains," and can be brought on by oxytocin releasing activities such as breastfeeding. There are herbal remedies that seem to help with afterpains, which I'll discuss in section 4.7.

Normal bleeding, similar to that of a regular menstrual cycle, will continue for about a week following birth.

The process by which the uterus returns to its non-pregnant size following childbirth is called involution. Uterine involution takes a full six weeks, but any noticeable contractions and afterpains should let up within three or four days after birth. Pee often during this period – a full bladder will displace the uterus. Peeing often empties the bladder giving the uterus plenty of space to contract effectively.

Six weeks after birth, when the uterus has returned to its pre-pregnancy size, is when I consider the process of childbirth, and the entire childbearing cycle to be complete. During these six weeks, you will make a profound transition into motherhood. Some find this transition to be smooth, and some find it rough. Nurture yourself as best as you are able during this time. Find help, wherever you can find it, in preparing meals, cleaning the house, food shopping, and taking care of younger children. Take this time to rest and bond with your newborn in whatever way seems right to you – these weeks are formative not only for your child, but also for yourself.

Atypical Presentations

A baby's presentation in-utero and as she moves through the birth canal can have an effect on both the length of labor and the mother's experience of labor and delivery. The *classic* optimal fetal presentations for a fast labor and easy delivery are called "occiput anterior" and "left occiput anterior." These presentations involve baby head-down and settled into the pelvis with her back to the mothers belly or with her back on the mother's left side. However, although these positions may be optimal most of the time, it does *not* mean that a different position would be anything less than optimal in an individual case. Every mother and every baby is different, and the natural intelligence of both bodies is at work when a baby chooses to birth "breech" or posterior.

The classic optimal fetal positions, Occiput Anterior (OA) and Left Occiput Anterior (LOA,) are the most common presentations in late pregnancy, occurring in the vast majority of natural labors. (It is often easy to tell when your baby is in one of these positions close to term. If your baby is OA, her back will be against your belly and there will be no kicking against your belly but rather gently movements and sliding. If your baby is LOA, her back and buttocks will be under your left ribs and will create a bulge, and you may often feel clear kicks under your right ribs.)

Other presentations, although not nearly as common, do occur in many births. These presentations are sometimes called "mal-presentations" because they may not provide an optimally-shaped pelvic opening to the presenting fetus during labor. However, the term "malpresentation" suggests that the presentations are poor or inferior, which is not always the case. Because of this, I prefer to call these presentations 'atypical' instead.

Two common types of atypical presentations include Breech ("bottom first,") and Posterior ("sunny side up" or "face up,") and two less common atypical presentations include Face and Brow. Breech and Posterior babies frequently result in a longer labor (although not always by any means,) as do babies presenting with their face (one in 500 births) or brow (one in 2,000 births.) All of these presentations can and often do, when left unhindered, result in normal delivery. These presentations present nuances to labor and delivery that differ from the average vertex (head-first, chin tucked, & rear-facing) baby, but through heeding bodily instincts and impulses, the mother can ease her baby's passage and safely deliver her baby.

Sometimes, babies choose to present in a certain atypical way and won't turn, no matter what. If the baby is in a position deemed a "variant of normal," then you can assume in these cases that the baby has a good reason to choose this position. Some women's bodies may simply be better suited to deliver a baby in an atypical position.

Other times, the baby assumes an atypical position not because it is *his* optimal position, but due to necessity of circumstances: lack of sufficient movement from the mother & a sedentary lifestyle, benign uterine tumors or 'fibroids,' nutritional deficiencies, or a number of other reasons can all cause a baby to assume a sub-optimal position. In these cases, lifestyle changes and gentle exercises during pregnancy can help the baby to turn, and will likely have a beneficial impact on the mother's birthing experience.

There are many simple lifestyle choices that can support an optimal fetal position. Movement throughout pregnancy is essential. It helps in stimulating your baby to move and, in later pregnancy, to engage in an optimal position for childbirth. Make sure you are eating a nutritious diet and listening to all of your body's needs. Support your liver and lymphatic system with gentle tonic herbs, and reduce excessive estrogen levels in the body through diet, as excess estrogen can contribute to uterine fibroids. There are many exercises you can do to help your baby engage in an optimal fetal position. Excellent & resourceful information on all types of possible presentations, and on techniques to safely turn a baby, can be found at this website: www.spinningbabies.com.

Moxibustion, a technique from traditional Chinese medicine, has also been used to successfully turn babies. Moxibustion works like this: Moxa, (also known as mugwort,) is tightly rolled into a wand or stick and burned like a smudging stick. The burning mugwort is placed close to certain acupuncture points, and activates those points with the heat and smoke from the mugwort. In the case of fetal positioning, the point most often used is UB 67, which is located on the outer edge of both pinkie toes. UB 67 is known to activate the uterus and to stimulate fetal movement.

Communication with your own body and your baby is also essential if you would like her to turn.

Pain, Ecstasy, &Surrender

"It is not possible for a woman to give birth without feeling anything. But what she feels can be a great joy to her."

~ Frederick Leboyer

Many, many women experience pain in childbirth.

Many, many women experience ecstasy in childbirth.

Pain and ecstasy are not contrary to one another. It is possible to experience both simultaneously, as I did – as many do. I think the problem lies in a lack of satisfactory language to describe the experience of childbirth. It is so, so far removed from most of our day to day life experience that we simply do not have the right words to describe it.

The word pain is not the right word to describe what most women experience as the intensity of contractions, and yet, when we rely on language to illustrate our experience, many women do experience pain simply because they do not know what else to call it, or because that is what they are expecting.

In other cases, there is pain – true pain – the body's response to something not right. It is easy to experience true childbirth pain if instincts are ignored during labor or during the prenatal period. In many modern hospital births, women are subjected to sub-optimal conditions; labor is hindered by these conditions, thus causing true pain. Many women work desk jobs and spend much of their pregnancy seated in a chair; lack of adequate movement throughout pregnancy causes the baby to assume a position in the womb that is not optimal for birth, thus causing prolonged labor and, sometimes, very painful contractions. During labor, a woman may need to vomit or poop but feel inhibited in front of strangers or even family – this physical inhibition and fear stalls the birth process, causing true pain.

There are many situations in which a woman may experience true pain during labor, but if both the prenatal period and the birth process are truly uninhibited, left to flow by nature's design, then true pain should not exist.

In a normal, unhindered labor, what exists is a deep, concentrated energy – an intensity beyond words. The best way, and the only way to describe these experiences is through metaphor.

What some call labor pains, I call the crashing of thunderous waves through your body – the rumble and roar of a storm so close that you feel it reverberating in your bones. You are rocked by the elemental power of childbirth – brought to your knees as these waves wash over you, sweep you into their churning sea. The undulating, rising and falling tides – peace, a glimpse of blue sky amidst the grey clouds, and the immanent knowing that this calm is only the eye of the storm – for it will rage until your baby is in your arms.

When I was a child, I often found myself near the ocean, playing in sand dunes with my brother or my cousins as our parents sat together on the beach. We would play in the water for hours, play with the waves – we learned to dive into the waves at just the right moment so that they would wash us up, gently, onto the shore – we studied the water, learned the patterns of the waves without realizing what we were doing.

One day, the waves were bigger than usual. I remember wading into the ocean on that windy day, deeper and deeper until I was up to my chest. The air was salty, warm... I saw, a ways off, a big, big wave coming. It was coming quickly. I felt excited – this would be a good wave to ride! I prepared myself to dive with the wave, to let it carry me on its crest, but I jumped at the wrong moment – a little too late. I missed the crest of the wave, and instead was engulfed in the waves underbelly – the pulling, swirling force underneath the water. I was totally submerged, my body swirling and dragging against the sand underwater. The force of that wave was so powerful that it swept my bathing suit clean-off. When the wave passed, I was left standing naked, shocked and shaken by the immense power I had just felt.

My dance with that wave is etched in my memory – it has stayed with me for many, many years, because that was the first time I felt a hint – just an inkling – of the immeasurable power of the earth. I was surrendered, completely at the mercy of the wave, and I felt a passion there that I had never felt before.

The power of childbirth is like the power of that wave – it sweeps you into a dance – a dance that you cannot control – a dance that bends you and twists you, rocks you and sways you. It is such a powerful wave, one that will only recede in its own time. The best thing you can do – the only thing you can do – is to surrender.

If I had tried to fight that wave as a child – if I had struggled against the current, I would have exhausted myself, and for what? Instead, I let the wave carry me. I became soft, supple, and malleable. In that surrender I felt a power more beautiful and immense than I had ever felt before – the power of nature.

Fifteen years later, as a woman giving birth, I surrendered to an even greater power – for in surrendering to the power of childbirth I not only witnessed the supreme power of nature, but also my own strength – my own immense power. I witnessed again my ability to let my body be taken – to let myself become so soft and malleable that the waves of birthing energy crashed through me and found no bones – to hardness – no rigidity to break.

The oak and the willow give us an amazing metaphor as well. The oak tree is known to be strongand robust, but also rigid. A powerful storm will take down a branch, and sometimes a whole tree. Its strength cannot hold up, sometimes, to force. The willow, on the other hand, is light. It is bendable, soft, and malleable. When you see a willow, you do not think of strength, but in times of stress, the willow is stronger than the oak. In a storm, her branches bend – they flow with the wind and do not resist.

In childbirth, our bodies should bend, soft, like the willow. Strength is needed to birth a child, but it is not a rigid strength – it is not about force or effort. It is about the strength to surrender – the strength to let go.

Pain comes when we fight against the current.

Pain comes when we are too rigid to bear the weight of the storm.

The strength needed in childbirth is the strength to change, to soften – the strength to let our bodies flow and ride with the power of life.

In the same way that the word pain does no justice in describing the waves of intense energy that churn your body throughout labor, neither do the words "ecstasy" and "bliss" to the immense joy that is felt throughout labor. In childbirth, the body is energized in a new way – there is a potent, real, present force. Your eyes are dilated – your cervix is dilated – your body, heart, soul, and your experience as a whole are open to the flow of life in a way never before felt.

The idea of experiencing pain in childbirth causes women to do many crazy things – to sign up for unnecessary medical procedures, C-sections, epidurals... This anxiety over pre-conceived pain compels so many women to deny themselves this powerful rite of passage – this inimitable journey into motherhood.

For those of you who have experienced trauma and immeasurable pain in childbirth, I am not denying this. I have heard this pain, wrenching screams – seen it, twisted expressions of agony. For you, perhaps you have felt the deeper, darker side to what I speak of – the deep and unforgivable power of nature.

Birth is not inherently painful. It is not a punishment for original sin. It is not a flaw of nature.

Pain comes when there is resistance, or when there is something wrong.

Truly unhindered birth is birth without resistance; unhindered birth comes through learning to meet your body's needs throughout pregnancy, learning to listen to your baby... it comes through learning to identify when things are not right, and finding solutions. It comes through learning to identify your inner voice, and respecting that voice as your greatest authority.

Truly unhindered birth is potent, intense, and ecstatic, but not painful.

"I flow with the waves and loose myself in them. I am ready, I open myself, I fall into ecstasy, and then, finally free, I let myself loose into eternity."

~ Letter from Marie G. Athens to Frederick Leboyer

Breath & Sound

Breath holds a great deal of power over your body, and can have profound effects on relaxation and the experience of childbirth. Many childbirth education classes teach breathing techniques to women in preparation for labor.

You can feel the effects of breath if you do a bit of experimentation. First, try taking a series of short, high, rapid breaths. Do not let the breath sink below your chest plate. How does this feel in your body?

Next, try taking one long, slow, deep breath. Do not over-inflate your lungs, but let the breath sink deep into your abdomen, into your womb, and down, even deeper, into your legs and feet. How does this feel in your body?

During labor, breathe down into your womb – into the earth. You don't have to breathe 'deep' as long as you breathe down – let the energy of your breath carry you down, loosen you – carry your baby down. When you breathe out, let your body sink and relax into the ground. Let your body open, and your baby descend. Combining breath with visualization in labor can be very helpful. Visualize opening, relaxing, releasing. Visualize your baby moving down through your open cervix, descending steadily through your birth canal and into your wide open arms.

When you combine breath with sound, it can have very profound effects. Low, deep chanting on the exhalation of a breath during labor can be very, very empowering. Deep sounds have the ability to send you deeper, to open you further, and to fully relax your body. When the sounds come from you, you can feel them reverberating throughout your body and changing your experience and the way you hold yourself. This is why, if you see a woman giving birth in ecstasy, you might hear her making those low moans, almost as though she is making love. Her body knows intuitively the power of sound.

If you feel inspired, you can practice these deep chanting sounds before labor begins; have the sound come from deep in your belly, through an unrestricted passage and out through a fully relaxed and open mouth. Making the sounds should not require any effort or cause any tension; rather, the sounds should totally relax you and dispel tension. It is not as much about how the sounds sound, not about the sounds being pretty or alluring – it is about how the sounds make you feel. They should make you feel primal, passionate, and deeply connected to your body's wisdom.

In many ways, childbirth is like having an incredibly intense bowel movement. The same opening and relaxation methods, although to a much milder degree, are required to poop as are required to birth a child. With this in mind, you can practice different breathing methods and sound techniques on the toilet each time you poop. This is a really good way to experiment with breath and sound before labor begins, and can help you to have an idea of what really works and what doesn't work for you. Maybe, for some, a bit of real pushing at the right moment after an inhalation could work miracles – for others, this may only prevent relaxation and hinder the processes.

Try different things if you feel called to experiment, and see what happens, but don't let this chapter narrow your view of the way birth needs to happen. For some women, thinking too much into breath can be a distraction. For some, this chapter may be totally unnecessary, for, in the end, your body knows just how to breathe to birth your baby.

Birth Positions & Practices

"I really wanted to get out of the birthing pool, and yet because I knew my friend and partner were into waterbirths, I felt uncomfortable owning this bodily need.... My mind kept me under rigid control for about half an hour, not being able to own my body's desire until it reached a critical point and my body almost threw me out of the birthing pool.... I walked up and down the stairs a few times, making loud primal noises whilst bearing down, intuitively and naturally, when I reached a contraction.... Then, almost out of nowhere, I felt an intense wave of energy course through my body, directing me into an even more aligned position ready for the baby to come out."

~ from "Jack's Unassisted Birth" written by Amelia Curtis, published in Veronika Robinson's "The Birthkeepers".

Positions

Walking and Standing – Walking is a wonderful and effective birth position. Mothers with slow contractions or prolonged labors may find that walking stimulates stronger, more effective contractions. Walking is a very good way to start labor. In Ina May's "Spiritual Midwifery," many of the birth stories start something like this: 'I went into labor. I called Ina May to tell her that the baby was coming, and she told me to go take walk and see how I felt after.'

Walking and standing are perfect positions during labor – they keep the baby engaged effectively in the pelvis, harness the power of gravity during contractions, and help the baby descend during the second stage.

Squatting – The squatting position can greatly increase the diameter of the pelvis, giving the baby more room to rotate in the birth canal and pass through the pelvis. Squatting decreases the likelihood of fetal asphyxiation, helps align the baby well with the mother's pelvis, and leaves room for the coccyx (tailbone) to move out of the way as the baby passes through the vagina. Many women feel the urge to assume this or a similar position during childbirth, and find that it makes contractions easier and quickens the progress of every stage of labor.

The squatting position was favored in many traditional cultures as an ideal position for giving birth. If you look at ancient sculptures and artifacts depicting our female ancestors giving birth, they are almost always in the squatting, kneeling, or "supported squat" positions.

Unlike today, squatting was integrated into the daily lives of our ancestors. They led a physically demanding lifestyle, and squatting was a part of almost every activity. Today, with chairs and tables, counters and refrigerators, cars, toilets, etc., we don't often have a need to squat and therefore our muscles aren't as accustomed to this exercise. Because of this, many women find squatting to be an uncomfortable position simply because their muscles aren't used to it.

There are many ways that to find support during a squat that turn it into a very comfortable and workable position. Leaning forward while squatting and supporting your weight with your hands touching the ground, or leaning backwards, with knees still tight to the chest, and being held or supported from behind by your partner or friends, are both helpful and carry all the same benefits of the squatting position.

Sitting – Sitting can be an effective position for labor. Many women feel that sitting on a toilet or a birthing chair help them to relax, as this is an environment where they are used to releasing their pelvic muscles. Sitting uses the force of gravity well, but may put pressure on the coccyx (tailbone) and immobilize it, making the final stages of labor more difficult.

Hands & Knees – The "hands and knees" position carries many of the same benefits as squatting – it widens the pelvic opening, quickens the progress of labor, makes fetal distress and asphyxia less likely, and is especially helpful in avoiding perennial tears.

This position can be very helpful for mothers experiencing long labors, especially if the baby is posterior, as it takes pressure off the back. This is also the 'go to' position if a baby's shoulders become stuck.

The 'hands and knees' position also includes positions where the mother is on her knees leaning over and resting on an object in front of her – a yoga ball, a bed or couch, or a birth partner. During the birth of my daughter, my body encouraged me to assume the 'hands and knees' position, with my front end draped over the seat of our couch, during almost every contraction. When I was starting to get tired, I would lay on my side on the couch, but as soon as a contraction came my body would almost force me out of the side-lying position and back onto my hands and knees. For some reason, this is how my daughter wanted to be born!

My son asked me to assume this position at the very end of my labor with him – just as he entered the birth canal. Before his birth I would have assumed that the 'hands and knees' position would not be a good way to catch your own baby, but I was alone at that birth and somehow I managed to catch Micah, one handed, as he slid out behind me!

Lying Down on the Back – Lying on the back became a standard practice for birthing mothers around the time that male doctors came into the birth picture. According to Lauren Dundes, author of "The Manner Born: Birth Rites in Cross-cultural Perspective," this position, also called the 'dorsal,' (or, with legs raised, the 'lithotomy') position, has early roots in France over 300 years ago. This position evolved because it allowed obstetricians easy access to the mother's vagina and her emerging baby. Its evolution had nothing whatsoever to do with the mother's or her baby's safety. In actuality, it is the worst position to give birth and should be completely avoided during labor.

The dorsal and lithotomy positions compress the uterus and partially cut off blood flow to the baby. These positions lengthen labor, increase the chance of fetal distress and asphyxia, increase the likelihood of perineal tears, narrow the pelvis and the birth canal, and are known to increase the chances of necessary medical intervention.

Side lying – Laying on the side is a good position for a mother to assume during labor if she is tired and in need of rest. It does not compress the uterus or restrict blood flow, as the dorsal position does, and can be helpful in-between contractions. I fell asleep in this position during the birth of my daughter, and am very grateful for the rest and strength it provided.

Practices to Facilitate Birth

Swaying, Rocking, and Jiggling – Birth is a dance. Hip rotation, swaying, rocking, and any constant movement all tend to speed labor and facilitate an easier passage for the baby. In some cultures, it was common for birth attendants to rub and jiggle the mother's legs and abdomen during the birth process. This helps to relax the mother's muscles and helps the baby move down.

All throughout my son's pregnancy I felt the urge to gently jiggle my belly. I would often do this subconsciously, and my partner seemed to think it was funny when he caught me doing it absentmindedly. I think there was a reason for this – my theory is that it helped me to relax my abdominal muscles and therefore helped Micah to maneuver inside of me and find his ideal birth position. When I went into labor with Micah, I found myself jiggling my belly through almost all of my early contractions. This helped in the same way during labor – it relaxed my abdominal muscles and helped ease me through contractions.

Ropes & Other Support – Leverage can enhance any birth position. Leverage can take many forms: ropes, bars, tree branches, beams, friends, or your partner can all provide this sort of leverage. In some hospitals and birthing centers there is a labor bed attachment called a "birthing bar" which can be used in the same way. In some cultures, it was commonplace to tie a rope to the ceiling and use this to pull down on while bearing down during labor. Leverage, in whatever form, can increase the effectiveness of contractions and facilitate labor.

Water – Laboring or birthing in water has many benefits and can enhance the efficiency labor in many ways. Warm water is soothing, comforting, and can help the mother to deeply relax her entire body, which is essential in childbirth. Water also provides a sense of lightness, which helps ease movements between birth positions and can make contractions easier as well. Many say that waterbirth also helps to ease the transition from womb to world for the baby.

When labor began with my son's birth, I immediately felt the need to take a warm, relaxing bath. I spent about 30 minutes there, but after a while it began to feel too restrictive for the movements that my body wanted to make. It was a small bathtub, so large bathtubs might not pose this problem, and birthing pools should have plenty of room.

One of the most beautiful birth stories that I read while I was pregnant for the first time depicted a mother who gave birth in the ocean. This story stuck with me – it's not something I would do – it seems too exposed – but it illustrated the fact that water birth is not limited to birthing pools and bath tubs.

There are no official accounts of traditional cultures birthing in water, but there are some incredibly beautiful legends depicting women laboring in tide pools, rivers and seas.

Your body has an innate knowledge, and will direct itself. It does not need forethought, or planning, or beliefs about which birthing positions or methods are better than others. I have included this list of birth positions & methods because I find the history, cultural differences, and modern practices of birth positions to be interesting and inspiring.

In labor, it is hard or even impossible to deny your impulses, as the quote at the beginning of this chapter illustrates. Trust that your body knows what is best for you. Don't get stuck, physically or mentally, in a certain position. Labor is most effective when you are active – actively listening and responding to your body's cues – moving, swaying, and engaging in this dance with your infant as she moves through you

Hormones during Childbirth

"Giving birth in ecstasy: This is our birthright and our body's intent. Mother Nature, in her wisdom, prescribes birthing hormones that take us outside (ec) our usual state (stasis), so that we can be transformed on every level as we enter motherhood. This exquisite hormonal orchestration unfolds optimally when birth is undisturbed, enhancing safety for both mother and baby."

~Sarah Buckley

The hormonal activity during the process of giving birth is amazing, and, in truth completely beyond the scope of rational human understanding.

Understanding the hormones of birth, of course, is not necessary for birth to unravel as nature intended, but learning about the hormones of birth is incredibly interesting and revealing. Even a basic comprehension of these hormones can reveal why some women feel pain during labor, and some only feel something that distantly resembles pain – why some women experience orgasmic, ecstatic births while some experience traumatic births.

Hormones are, in essence, the messengers of our bodies – they carry information from one place to another in a single body, and also from one body to another. Humans have only the faintest glimpse into the complexities of the hormone systems of the body, and in my opinion that glimpse is enough to know that the entire human body has an incredible, unfathomable innate intelligence.

This chapter gives a glimpse into that intelligence – a very rudimentary overview which, in truth, does absolutely no justice to the simultaneously indescribably complex and beautifully simple process of childbirth. Trying to describe childbirth with humanity's understanding of hormones is like trying to describe the experience of beautiful music with the science of the ear. It is, in many ways, completely futile. Still, I find this rudimentary understanding to be interesting and somewhat enlightening, so I will share it here all the same.

There are four major hormone groups that play an active role during labor: oxytocin, beta-endorphins, catecholamines, and prolactin. There are also two that play a role in the onset of labor: estrogen and progesterone.

Estrogen and Progesterone: Estrogen and progesterone prepare the body for labor; according to Chris Kresser, "estrogen has… been shown to increase the number of uterine oxytocin receptors and gap junctions in late pregnancy, which is thought to prepare the uterus for contractions in labor." These hormones prepare other hormonal systems, and set the stage for childbirth.

Oxytocin: Oxytocin is the hormone of love, affection, and selfless giving. Besides its role in the birth process, oxytocin also plays a crucial part in sex, orgasm, and breastfeeding, and also in non-reproductive loving situations, like simply spending time with family or close friends.

Oxytocin governs the regularity of contractions, and peaks as your baby is crowning, stimulated by receptors that are triggered as your vagina stretches. This peak lasts until after the birth of the placenta.

Beta-endorphins: Beta-endorphins are responsible for pleasure and ecstasy. These hormones are released from the pituitary gland during times of pain, and activate a pleasurable response from the body to produce a feeling of joy, ecstasy, and satisfaction in the birth process.

Beta-endorphins produce a euphoric trance which many women experience during birth. This trance is ecstatic, and completely diminishes any feeling of pain. If these hormones are inhibited during labor, which they can be in many modern birth situations, then birth loses much of its magic and becomes painful.

Beta-endorphins also set the stage for prolactin release during labor.

Catecholamines: Catecholamines are stress hormones – they include adrenaline and noradrenaline, and are the hormones responsible for the "fight or flight" response.

These hormones play a very interesting role in birth. If they are activated too early or through any external fear-inducing circumstances, these hormones can slow or stop labor. However, according to Sarah Buckley, these hormones play a role in the transition from the first stage to the second stage of labor:

> *"When the moment of birth is imminent... there is a sudden increase in CA levels, especially noradrenaline, which activates the fetal ejection reflex. The mother experiences a sudden rush of energy; she will be upright and alert, with a dry mouth and shallow breathing and perhaps the urge to grasp something. She may express fear, anger, or excitement, and the CA rush will cause several very strong contractions, which will birth the baby quickly and easily."*

> *~Sarah Buckley*

It is hard to say what causes what, in this case. This sudden rush of catecholamines may be why some women suddenly feel fear or stress as they pass into transition – because they are experiencing a sudden great rush of tremendously intense energy. Alternatively, it may be that stress or fear felt nearing the moment of transition is the trigger for this sudden release of catecholamines, meaning that stress at this point in labor is actually necessary to facilitate an effective second stage.

Levels of catecholamines drop again immediately after birth. Their role is only to stimulate an enormous rush of energy after full cervical dilation which helps to push the baby out quickly and effectively. I remember this rush so clearly, as it happened in the transitional phasesduring the births of my son and second daughter. Coupled with the high levels of oxytocin and beta-endorphins at that time, there is no other ecstatic moment in my life that I can say compares to that!

Prolactin – Prolactin is known as the mothering hormone. It actually decreases during labor but rises suddenly at the time of birth. Prolactin, along with oxytocin, is responsible for the unselfish giving of mothers to their infant's needs. As the name suggests, prolactin plays a major role in breastfeeding.

~*~

"Spontaneous labour in a normal woman is an event marked by a number of processes so complicated and so perfectly attuned to each other that any interference will only detract from the optimal character."

~ G. Kloosterman

Disruption or manipulation of the unique and intricate hormonal process is both completely unnecessary and detrimental to both mother and child. The operation of these hormones during labor depends greatly on the environment of the birth and the attitude of the mother. Without fear, stress, manipulation, or intervention, these hormones flow perfectly and conduct the body perfectly, like an elaborate and exquisite symphony. The body must be willing to listen to the cues of the conductor, and the environment should be conducive to the conductor's visibility in the first place. In order for the environment to be conducive in this way, one must create an atmosphere which is least obstructive to the systems in the brain which are responsible for our hormonal orchestration.

The pituitary gland and hypothalamus, which are responsible for hormonal orchestration during labor, are part of the limbic brain, also known as the mammalian brain. When prompted by the hypothalamus, hormones are released directly into the bloodstream from the pituitary gland. Oxytocin, for example, is released in rhythmic pulses from the pituitary gland during labor. The pulses of oxytocin become closer and closer together as labor progresses. This is what contributes to the regularity and increasingly close intervals of contractions during the birth process.

The functioning of the limbic brainis influenced greatly by our environment. The limbic brain operates best when certain parts of the neocortex are not highly activated. Social processing and inhibition are associated with the neocortex, as is language processing.

The increase in the complexity and size of the human neocortex in human evolution marked an increase in social inhibition, which was beneficial because it produced greater social harmony. However although social harmony may be beneficial for our species as a whole, social inhibition has negative implications for individuals. An environment which does not stimulate these processing centers in the neocortex is conducive to the optimal functioning of the limbic brain and hormonal progression and is therefore conducive to a smooth, unhindered labor. How could we create such an environment?

Regular monitoring, whether technical or non-technical, can wrench the mother out of her intuitive limbic brain and into these centers of theneocortex. Progress, or lack-thereof, is a concept that can only be rationalized in the neocortex.In this way, monitoring inhibits intuition and the hormonal process necessary for unhindered childbirth.

Talking, which seems simple and non-problematic, can suppress optimal functioning of the limbic brain. If there is too much talk – conversation, questions, comments around the mother as she is giving birth, this could affect her hormonal process by over-stimulating the language processing center of the neocortex. If possible, details should be worked out beforehand so that all people involved know their role in the birth, making the use of language less necessary during the birth itself. If language is necessary, it can be direct and brief – a call to action ("Get water." or "Stand here, support me.") or a statement ("No more." or "That helps.")

Dim lighting is also favorable, since bright lighting can make us feel more exposed – more visible to others. – In bright light, there is a greater likelihood of activating the social processing center of the neocortex due to that feeling of exposure. Dim lighting provides a feeling of concealment, making social inhibition less likely.

During my births, I found that I had very little need (or ability) to use complex language – my focus was so internal and my bodily needs so clear, that it made the use of language almost unnecessary. Joey seemed to intuitively understand this, especially in my third birth, and when I wanted him to be there with me for support, he sat quietly until I asked something of him. He got me water when I said "water", understood simple gestures as calls to action, and was able to keep his extraneous thoughts to himself. Afterwards, he told me he had been thinking all sorts of things that I really wouldn't have wanted to hear or process during the birth.

My least socially inhibited moment of birth was when I was completely alone during the last 15 minutes of the birth of my son. Birth flowed so optimally during that time. I noticed that I was quieter, even though the contractions were very intense, than I was during the pushing phases of my other two births. It is almost as if the vocalizations of intensity were only necessary for me in a social setting. Our brain and the processes of our bodies are so complex and interesting.

"For birth to proceed optimally, [the mammalian brain] must take precedence over the neocortex, or rational brain. This shift can be helped by an atmosphere of quiet and privacy with, for example, dim lighting and little conversation, and no expectation of rationality from the laboring woman. Under such conditions a woman will intuitively choose the movements, sounds, breathing, and positions that will birth her baby most easily. This is her genetic and hormonal blueprint."

~ Sarah Buckley

Herbs for Childbirth

The process of childbirth is totally, completely, and utterly natural. Herbs are certainly not essential during childbirth. Many herbs, however, may be of help in certain unusual situations. The following chapter is not meant to suggest that any of these herbs are necessary to facilitate childbirth – unhindered childbirth requires nothing but a safe space and a relaxed & healthy mother. Using herbs unnecessarily is not only pointless, but is also potentially detrimental.

Many women, however, choose to prepare for childbirth by having some herbs on hand just in case the birth is not progressing as expected. Having herbs on hand for childbirth is prudent; using herbs without a clear reason is not.

I suggest that you read through the following chapter, and take note of any herbs that stand out to you. Have any herbs on hand that you feel may be helpful for you during labor. Do what makes you feel comfortable and safe. Read the dosages, instructions for use, and precautions carefully, and further familiarize yourself with any herb you intend to use before labor begins.

I had a few herbs on hand, but did not use any during my first two births. With my third labor, I did use shepherd's purse tincture when my bleeding seemed heavy after the placenta came. I also used motherwort liberally to help me cope with the afterpains, which were much stronger than they had been with my first two births.

"Any type of intervention is an intervention.... If a mother wants to use herbal remedies in labor, they can be a great alternative to pharmaceutical drugs, with appropriate usage and education.... As an herbalist, I am wary of herbal practices that mimic modern medicine. Herbs should not be used to be used. I also do not believe in starting herbs to assist labor five weeks beforehand. Babies are born, without herbs and without drugs, every day."

~ Demetria Clark

Herbs for the 1st & 2nd stages of Labor

Motherwort – Motherwort has a beautifully relaxing effect on the nerves. It is a uterine tonic, as well as a great ally to the heart. The Latin name, Leonurus cardiaca, literally means "lion-hearted." Motherwort can instill grace and courage; it is like the little mother – supporting, nurturing, and soothing. Motherwort is an amazing ally to all women, but has a special affinity for mothers.

Some women take a few drops of motherwort tincture, coupled with red raspberry leaf infusion and Partridge Berry tea, daily in the last few weeks of pregnancy to tone the uterus in preparation for childbirth.

Motherwort also shines immediately after the birth of your child, which I'll discuss below in "herbs for the 3rd stage of labor," and throughout the entire journey of motherhood.

During the 1st stage of labor, a few drops of motherwort tincture under the tongue or in a glass of water can help to relax, soothe, and center the birthing mother, and can instill courage and dispel anxiety and fear. The suggested dose is 5 drops of tincture every few hours. The effects if used under the tongue will come on more rapidly and disperse more quickly; the effects if used in a small glass of water will come on a little slower but will last longer, usually up to three hours.

Susun Weed suggests that motherwort is contraindicated if contractions are irregular, as it can produce a "floating or non-existent feeling in the uterus."

Motherwort tincture is much more potent when it has been made with fresh, rather than dried herb. I've had trouble finding commercially available motherwort tincture that's been made with fresh herb, so you would probably have better luck making it yourself or sourcing it from an independent herbalist or a small, local company.

Blue Cohosh – Blue cohosh root is widely renowned as an herb for labor. Many midwives include the tincture of blue cohosh in their birth kits. It can initiate labor, help keep contractions strong and regular, tone the uterus, and ease delivery.

Blue cohosh should only be used to initiate labor if there is a good, clear reason for doing so, such as premature rupture of membranes with no labor in sight. The dose of tincture to initiate labor, according to Susun Weed, is *"3-8 drops in a glass of warm water or tea.... Repeat every half hour for several hours until contractions are regular. If labor is not underway in four hours, use a dropperful of the tincture under the tongue every hour for up to four more hours or until contractions are strong and consistent."* (Remember that for labor to begin successfully, the cervix must be soft and ready. This is called a "ripe cervix." Making love, especially if the woman reaches orgasm, is known to soften the cervix, but should not be attempted if the membranes have ruptured. Black cohosh can also be used to ripen the cervix.)

To speed or encourage a stalled labor, the dose of blue cohosh tincture is 10 to 20 drops hourly for up to 8 hours.

Many use blue and black Cohosh in combination. According to Susun Weed, "they seem to work better together than alone, a synergistic pair producing regular and coordinated contractions."

Black Cohosh – Black cohosh is often used in combination with blue cohosh to initiate labor. It has a softening effect on the cervix. The dose is 10 drops of tincture, directly in the mouth, hourly. According to Susun Weed, this should have a very noticeable effect on the cervix within three or four hours.

Black cohosh can also be used to relieve muscle pain and spasms. It can be used as a liniment, (a tincture applied externally to painful areas,) or taken internally to relieve pain.

Some midwives suggest using black cohosh in the weeks before labor begins to tone the uterus or to ensure that the baby is born at term. I do not believe this would be necessary, and feel it could be detrimental. I believe birth happens in its own time. I suggest doing some thorough research into this method before employing it.

Lobelia – Lobelia is relaxing to the body's musculature and very helpful during labor for its ability to dispel rigidity. It is especially helpful if the cervix is soft but rigid, that is, ripe but not dilating. Lobelia is a controversial herb – considered unsafe by many. For some people, it can cause nausea and vomiting or a trance-like state.

Still, according to Susun Weed it is recommended by many herbalists and midwives for *"rigid o's, uteri with rigid rim, [and] perineal and vaginal rigidity in labor.... The effect is transitory, rarely lasting more than 30 minutes.... A sufficiently large dose will usually cause some strange sensations such as a tingling in the extremities, flushing, and a rubbery feeling in the face. Smaller doses will increase nervous energy, talkativeness, and lighten the mood."*

Some people report that very long labors can successfully come to a conclusion within an hour or two of using Lobelia tincture. In these cases, I would assume that there was some physical, mental, or emotional barrier to relaxing and opening during labor.

Use lobelia during labor only if necessary. Some suggest a dropperful every hour if you are having problems relaxing and opening during labor; others suggest a dose as often as every 30 minutes until relaxation is sufficient for labor to progress. Susun Weed suggests a large dose: "60-150 drops... in a quarter glass of water. The dose may be repeated two times, at thirty minute intervals, or until the o's relax." It is slightly unclear, but I believe she is suggesting no more than three total doses. I would also suggest using a smaller amount first to gage your individual reaction to lobelia.

Bethroot – Bethroot, also known as birthroot and trillium, can be used to initiate a stalled labor. Trillium is very rare, and is endangered in many states. It is one of my favorite flowers to happen upon in the woods in spring, so I do not feel it is wiseto misuse or overuse this beautiful plant. Bethroot was used by Native Americans to induce and strengthen contractions, ensure an easy delivery, and decrease the likelihood of post-partum hemorrhage. In her "Wise Women Herbal for the Childbearing Year," Susun Weed writes that "one pregnant midwife reports chewing the raw root of Trillium to start her labor and having immediate contractions."

If you choose to use bethroot, Susun Weed's standard dose of tincture is "1/4 to ½ teaspoon" at "thirty minute intervals," and this dose should not be taken for more than a total of three times.

Cannabis – Cannabis is one of humanity's most widely known and loved herbal allies. Perhaps all too often it is misused or abused, but it has much to offer as an herbal medicine.

A very small amount of Cannabis, smoked or used as a tincture, can help facilitate a stalled labor. Cannabis is oxytocic, and can be a great ally for releasing emotional or mental tension that may be hindering the birth process.

Cannabis is illegal in many states. I would not suggest using this herb during birth unless there is a good reason, such as stalled or prolonged labor. If you have never used cannabis before, I do not suggest that you use it for the first time while giving birth, as the herb has a powerful effect on some people and can even cause anxiety and paranoia if used in too high a dose. If you are comfortable using cannabis and know how dosage affects you, however, it may be a great ally during the birth process. Susun weed describes the effects of cannabis during childbirth as 'magnifying.' "*It will magnify what is in the room, in the psychic air, in the emotional aura, in the birthing woman, in the sensory field. This magnification, used wisely, is of tremendous aid to both midwife and birthing woman, heightening their connection to and responsiveness to the baby being born.*" Susun weed warns, though, that if used in an atmosphere of fear, anger or uncertainty, cannabis will magnify those qualities, having a stronglydetrimental effect on the progress of labor.

Cotton Root Bark – Cotton root bark has a great reputation, in the American south and other places where it was traditionally grown, as an herb to promote strong, effective contractions and to speed labor. It is especially helpful for prolonged or irregular labors. Susun Weed suggests drinking sips of a strong infusion of the root bark to stimulate labor. It can also be taken in tincture form.

Cotton root bark should never be used during pregnancy, since its powerful uterine stimulating properties can cause abortion or miscarriage.

Make sure, if you use cotton root bark, that it is sourced from organically grown cotton. Non-organic cotton is usually laden with toxic pesticides.

Hops – Hops tea, sipped slowly, can be an effective remedy for high blood pressure during labor. According to Susun Weed, this tea can be made more effective if "10-20 drops of each Skullcap and Valerian tinctures" are added to it. Hops, the same herb used in many beers, is very relaxing. Some women report that sipping a small amount, (8oz or less, depending on body weight,) of beer during labor induces mild muscle relaxation and helps facilitate labor.

Raspberry Leaf – Raspberry leaf is not only an amazing tonic herb for use during pregnancy – it can also help to gently tone the uterus and facilitate contractions during labor.

Many women prepare for labor by making a strong raspberry leaf infusion and freezing it in an ice cube tray. They take the tea-cubes out of the freezer once labor begins, and suck on them throughout the entire childbirth process.

The effects of Raspberry are cumulative: it is a tonic. For best results, use raspberry leaf infusion weekly throughout your entire pregnancy, or at the very least, in the last month before birth.

Herbs for the 3rd Stage of Labor

Motherwort – Motherwort is soothing, calming, and a beautiful herb to have on hand immediately after childbirth. It helps to center and relax the mother, and is also known to prevent postpartum hemorrhage. Susun Weed writes that "midwives who give 10 drops of Motherwort tincture to every mother after the baby is born claim that it totally prevents hemorrhage." (For more on motherwort, see the section on "Herbs for the 1st and 2nd Stages of Labor.") Motherwort tincture can be taken immediately after your baby's birth as hemorrhage prevention.

Raspberry Leaf – Raspberry leaf infusion continues to gently strengthen the uterus after the birth, facilitating continued contractions and the birth of the placenta, and making hemorrhage less likely. Raspberry leaf works very gently and has a tonic effect, and should not be used in cases of acute hemorrhage or retained placenta. Raspberry leaf infusion can be made into ice cubes before labor begins, and then sucked on any time during labor as desired.

Ground Ivy – Ground Ivy herb has been used historically to prevent a retained placenta. According to Susun Weed, a standard dose is a cup of infusion or ½ to 1 teaspoon of the tincture of "*Glechoma hederacea*" immediately after birth.

Angelica or Dong Quai – Angelica can be used in acute cases of a retained placenta. Susun Weed suggests that a 30 to 50 drop dose of the tincture will almost always work to stimulate the uterus to expel the placenta within minutes. Angelica is a powerful herb and should always be used with respect.

Blue Cohosh – Blue cohosh can be used in the 3rd stage of labor to facilitate continued & effective contractions. It can be used in conjunction with angelica to help deliver a retained placenta if there is heavy bleeding. Neither of these herbs should be used as a preventative – only in cases where contractions have slowed or stopped, leading to retained placenta and heavy bleeding. According to Susun Weed, a dose is 20 drops of tincture repeated "in 2-5 minutes, if necessary."

Witch Hazel – Witch hazel is known for its powerfully astringent properties. If bleeding is distressingly heavy and the placenta has not yet been delivered, Witch hazel tincture and can be used to control bleeding. The dose is 10 to 20 drops, as needed.

Shepherd's Purse – Shepherd's purse is one of the most well-known herbs for stopping a postpartum hemorrhage. Not only does it help the blood to form clots, quickly stemming the flow of a hemorrhage, but it also promotes contractions which help the uterus to return to a smaller size, addressing the root cause of the hemorrhage.

Shepherd's Purse should not be used until after the placenta and all afterbirth has been delivered. A dose is one full dropper of tincture taken directly under the tongue. According to Susun Weed, "thirty seconds is the longest any midwife has reported it taking to significantly slow or completely stop bleeding." Teas and infusions of dried shepherd's purse are not effective, as the herb loses most of its potency in the drying process. Susun also cautions that tinctures made from the dried herb are not nearly as potent as tinctures made from the fresh herb. She suggests making your own tincture from fresh plants in the springtime, or buying the tincture only from those who have crafted it using the fresh plant.

Lobelia – Lobelia can be used in cases of mild (or severe) shock, that is, dizziness, pallor of the skin, and general weakness following major blood loss if a hemorrhage cannot be stopped quickly enough. Susun Weed suggests "3 to 5 drops repeated every 5 minutes as needed." Severe shock is life-threatening.

Postpartum Wisdom

"A woman is the full circle. Within her is the power to create, nurture and transform."

~ *Diane Mariechild*

Stepping through the doorway to motherhood is an enormous transition. It is a rite of passage – an entrance into a new stage of feminine life. This passage is most profound when a woman crosses that doorstep for the first time, leaving her maidenhood behind and experiencing her new life as a mother.

This is a beautiful, light-filled, heavenly and sometimes tumultuous time. You are blessed with the presence of your newborn – blessed with the gift of her deep, new eyes – blessed with the opportunity to meet her, to know her, to call her by her name and love her more deeply than you ever knew was possible. With that said, you will probably also be sleep deprived. You may experience the transition of your pregnant to non-pregnant body to be somewhat uncomfortable. You may need help – lots of help.

In a way, in becoming a mother, you are given the gift of learning to surrender. The passage of childbirth teaches surrender; it is an initiation into the maternal world of surrender – of true and unfathomable joy in letting go – of selfless giving and unconditional love.

Some say that in becoming a mother, you are no longer the center of your universe. In a way, this is true; you are no longer alone at the center of your universe. In becoming a mother, you do not discard yourself – you do not abandon yourself for your children. Rather, in becoming a mother, you transform for your children; you shine in ways you never knew possible.

The process of childbirth is only the beginning! In motherhood, you discover your strength, your weakness, your beauty, your shadow, your compassion, and your thresholds. Each facet of your whole being evolves – transforms – blossoms. The passage of motherhood not only marks the birth of your child – it marks your own rebirth, as well.

Table of Contents for Postpartum Wisdom

Breastfeeding

*"It is only in the act of nursing that a woman realizes her
motherhood in visible and tangible fashion; it is a joy of
every moment."*

~ Honore de Balzac

The breastfeeding relationship is a beautifully symbolic image of the
mother-child relationship. It is a portrayal of the abundant giving and
surrender of motherhood. It represents love and nourishment
flowing from the mother into her child – a continuity of maternal
nourishment from the womb environment into the environment of
the larger world.

Culturally, newborns are imagined as helpless and devoid of
intelligence. They are seen as an open slate, needing to be trained and
guided in order to learn about the world. In many ways, perhaps, this
may be true, but it is not true of the relationship between a newborn
and his mother.

Babies, seconds old, have reflexes designed to initiate
breastfeeding. They are ready – they anticipate the task before them
and know how to accomplish it, if left to their own devices. If a
mother reclines on her back and places her newborn child on her
chest, skin to skin, the newborn will, without any assistance, locate,
latch on, and begin suckling on his mother's breast.

A 1990 film, "Delivery Self Attachment," by Dr. Lennart Righard
and Margaret Alade, documents newborn babies crawling up their
mothers' chests without assistance, finding their breasts, and initiating
breastfeeding without any assistance. In a 2003 article written by "La
Leche League" leader Teresa Pitman, one Canadian midwife was able
to witness this occurrence in some of her clients who had seen the
film and were interested in testing the theory.

Before reading this, I assumed that breastfeeding was something
that needed to be initiated by the mother. Had I known that infants
were capable of initiating breastfeeding before giving birth, I would

have let my children find their own ways to my breast. Perhaps that would have helped my daughter in her first few weeks of life.

When Peacy was born, she cried. She did not want to nurse, and cried herself to sleep. After sleeping, she still did not want to nurse. This lasted many hours, and it seemed like the more I offered my breast to her, the more she resisted.

I was worried that she was not getting enough nourishment. During that first week, her nursing was infrequent, agitated, and short-lived. My breasts became so engorged with colostrum that they hurt, and every night for about a week I would wake to find my sheets soaked with milk.

This evening, I stumbled upon Theresa Pitman's article "Infant Self-Attachment," which opened up a whole new world to me. Maybe, if I had stopped trying in increasing desperation to "help" Peacy to nurse, she would have eventually decided, in her own time, that she was ready. Rather than telling Peacy it was time to 'try again,' perhaps I should have waited for her to tell me she was ready and willing, even if that took hours, a day, or even two.

"A new mother called me.... Her baby boy, born uneventfully at home, was 12 hours old at this point and had still not taken the breast. When the mother and midwife tried to help him latch on, he closed his mouth firmly and arched his back, pulling his head away from the breast.... I suggested to the mother that she just concentrate for a little while on helping the baby feel relaxed and comfortable at the breast — just letting him lie there, close to the breast, without any pressure to latch on or feed. She called me back several hours later, very excited, with wonderful news. She had been lying on her back, dozing, with her naked baby lying on his stomach on her bare abdomen just below her breasts. She noticed the baby beginning to squirm and wriggle and then, to her surprise, he pushed himself up to her breasts, his little head bobbing as he searched for the nipple."

~ Theresa Pitman

Eventually Peacy established a normal pattern of nursing. My breasts caught on to her needs and made just the right amount of milk. I feel like Peacy and I could have avoided a lot of stress in those first few weeks, however, if I had trusted in the breastfeeding process as much as I trusted in the birth process.

Many babies latch on very soon after birth, and some wait. Some babies are eager to breastfeed, and some, like Peacy, are very resistant to the idea and just need some time.

Working with your Baby: Your baby has a few main reflexes that are involved in their innate knowledge of breastfeeding. Some of these reflexes are centered in the feet and limbs; if a baby's feet are stimulated when he is on his belly, he will make crawling movements with his legs. This, in theory, is to help him squirm and wriggle his way to the breast. Other of these reflexes are centered in the cheeks and mouth – if one of a baby's cheeks is touched or brushed with a finger, he will automatically turn in the direction of that cheek. This is called the rooting reflex, and often involves the baby bobbing his head rapidly from side to side, in search of a nipple. If his mouth makes contact with something he believes to be a nipple he will automatically begin sucking. Many babies mistake fingers, noses, and knuckles for nipples in their first few days of life.

Many women find that breastfeeding their infants is easy – that it is second nature. Others, however, find it to be much more difficult than they had imagined, or hoped. Many mothers give up breastfeeding because it is painful, because their infant will not latch on, or because they are not making sufficient milk. For the mothers who find breastfeeding to be effortless, nothing more is needed. For the others, who desire to breastfeed but find it very challenging, there may be steps you can take to ease the process, facilitating maternal instincts as well as neonatal reflexes that support simple, relaxed, painless and successful breastfeeding.

Suzanne Colson, a midwife and nurse, is the originator of "biological nurturing." Biological nurturing is a "new" approach to newborn bonding based on Suzanne's extensive explorations into the effects of maternal positioning on the mother-child relationship and breastfeeding.

Suzanne Colson and many others in the past decade have found that contrary to popular belief, human babies are not "dorsal feeders." That is, human infants are not designed to feed while lying on their backs; rather, they are designed to be abdominal feeders.

Optimal activation of a newborn's breastfeeding reflexes occurs when the mother is in a partially reclined, totally supported position. The mother should be at a comfortable angle supported by lots of pillows – pillows under her back, head, arms, etc., so that she can completely relax into a partially reclining position. The infant is placed on her mother's abdomen, facing her mother ('chest to belly' or 'chest to breast,' not 'back to arm,' etc.) and completely supported by gravity on the mother's chest. This stimulates instinctive action in both the mother and her child. The child is not asked to breastfeed, and is not even necessarily placed with her mouth near the nipple. Rather, the infant will signify, if and when she is ready, that she is interested in breastfeeding, and the mother instinctually helps, if needed.

"During BN, mother's shoulders, neck and head are supported while they gaze, groom and coo at their newborn. Each baby's unique behavioral response is usually the only breastfeeding instruction a mother needs."

~Suzanne Colson

Because of the positioning involved, Colson calls biological nurturing "the laid back breastfeeding revolution." The goal of biological nurturing is not only to stimulate breastfeeding, although that is often the result. It also serves as a means by which the mother and her newborn can acquaint themselves with one another in a comfortable, loving, intimate fashion.

Many mothers naturally assume this position with their infant in the hours or days after birth. It is instinctual. I felt this instinct after Peacy's birth, but denied it. At the time, we lived in a tiny log cabin. We slept on a fold-out bed which had no headboard. The interior walls of the cabin were white-washed, and the wash would come off in a dusty powder if they were brushed up against... It was all I wanted to do in those days after Peacy's birth to lean our only two pillows against the wall to make a comfortable and supported place for me to recline to feed her, but I declined that instinct because I did not want the white wash to crumble onto our only pillows and bed. In retrospect, I may have saved myself a lot of stress if I had let go of that concern and listened to my instincts.

Colson also stresses that a baby does not have to be awake to breastfeed. In fact, she says that biological nurturing is most effective when the baby is allowed to gently doze in this position. A sleepy, relaxed, and emotionally comfortable baby is more apt to latch on without resistance.

Of course, any position that works is a good position. Colson's techniques simply stand to offer a different, and possibly gentler and more comfortable, approach to breastfeeding and nurturing in those early days of your infants life.

Pumping, Colostrum, & Breast Engorgement: Many midwives and lactation experts suggest that if your newborn does not latch on within the first few hours of birth, you should begin expressing milk. This is suggested for a few reasons:

Firstly, colostrum, produced for the first few days following your baby's birth, is an incredibly healing and nourishing food for your baby. You should consider saving every ounce of colostrum that you make to spoon-feed or dropper-feed to your infant.

Secondly, expressing milk will keep your milk supply coming strong. Your body makes milk only as your child demands it. If your child is not breastfeeding for a few days, this could decrease your overall milk supply. Your supply can, of course, return full force if your baby begins nursing, but it may take a day or two to catch up to his needs.

Thirdly, pumping can help to prevent or alleviate breast engorgement, which is not only often painful, but also makes latching on even more difficult for your infant.

I have small nipples, and I found that expressing milk by hand was somewhat difficult for me. This is not the case for everyone, but if you have difficulty expressing by hand, there are both manual powered and electronic breast milk pumps available.

Thoughts on Bottle Feeding:I was in a store recently, buying fruit for my two older children, when we were all approached by a woman who said she was a nurse at our local hospital. My 5-month old was in a sling. She looked at my youngest and said, "She must be a breast baby!"

"Yes," I said. I was overwhelmed at being in the store in the first place, and really feeling like I just wanted to leave and get home.

The woman went on, "I can tell... she looks so content. She's smiling. I bet she never cries."

"She cries," I said.

"Oh," she went on, slightly surprised, "You're making the right choice..." I didn't know what to say, so I just said 'think you' and went to the checkout line, not really wanting to engage in a conversation at the time.

Point being: There are a lot of opinions out there, some full of judgment, but the only one who knows best is you. There is absolutely nothing wrong with choosing to bottle-feed your baby.

Breastfed babies cry. So do bottle fed babies. Crying is a baby's healthy and natural response to something not right – both breastfed and bottle fed babies perceive things as not right at times.

Although breastfeeding does have many benefits, including greater immune support for the baby, what is truly important is the bond created between mother and child; this bond can be accomplished through breastfeeding or bottle feeding. I chose to breastfeed my children because I absolutely love the experience. I love the easiness of it. I never have to worry about mixing formula or bringing it out with me – never have to wash bottles or freeze leftover milk. Wherever I am, my breasts are there too! And the way it feels when the milk is let down and the swelling of my breasts... I just love it. But some don't feel that way, and that is ok. It is more important to be honest with yourself about how you feel – more important to find workable ways to enjoy motherhood than it is to stick to an ideal. There are also many programs that I know of in the US and Canada dedicated to making (human) breast milk available to babies whose mothers are not able to breastfeed!

Herbs, Nutrition, & Lifestyle to Support Breastfeeding

Galactagogues

Galactagogues are herbs known to encourage a plentiful milk supply. They are best used in combination with plenty of rest and a healthy and calorie-dense diet.

Borage: Borage is one of my favorite herbs to grow, and has a well-deserved reputation for increasing milk supply. I love to see the seedlings emerge from the soil. I love to harvest the thick, juicy leaves when they are young and vibrant green to make a nourishing tea. The flowers are so beautiful and delicious. They melt in your mouth like little drops of sweet, cool rain. Borage tea is best made with the fresh mucilaginous leaves, as the dried leaved have lost most of their medicinal value. It is a soothing herb for the heart – a joyful friend and ally. Borage is my favorite herbal galactagogue. Some say to use caution with this herb during breastfeeding due to the possibility of potentially liver-damaging alkaloids that may be secreted in the milk. Borage and comfrey are related, and the same has been said of comfrey. Personally, I do not believe that borage poses any threat whatsoever when used as an occasional herbal tea, but do your own research and be your own authority on this matter.

Fenugreek: Fenugreek seed can be added to herbal tea or used in cooking, and is well known to increase milk supply. It has a beautifully sweet earthy smell, like maple syrup. I like it best in moderation, since in larger amounts it can taste bitter.

Blessed Thistle: A bitter herb with an affinity for postpartum women, this thistle increases milk supply and can help to relieve mild post-partum depression as well. Blessed Thistle also goes by the name of "Our Lady's Milk Thistle." ("Our lady's milk thistle"/"blessed thistle" and "milk thistle" are two different plants despite the similar name.) The infusion is very, very bitter; many women prefer the tincture. You can drink one or two cups of the infusion or use up to 80 drops of tincture every day.

Fennel (or Anise) Seed: Fennel seed is a delicious addition to herbal teas and cooking. I love the smell and the taste. It is a digestive aid, and encourages a strong flow of milk. Susan Weed suggests Fennel-Barley Tea, which is delicious & involves making an infusion of barley, straining the barley, bringing the barley water to a boil and then pouring the boiling water over the fennel seeds to steep for a short time – 10 to 30 minutes.

Shatavari: Although I've never personally used this herb to increase milk supply, it has a reputation as an effective galactagogue and I thought it was worth including. Shatavari is a traditional Woman's herb in Ayurvedic medicine. It is used to tone and strengthen the reproductive organs, to increase fertility, as a general female tonic. It is a relative of asparagus, and has a pleasant taste.

Catnip: Catnip Tea, when drank by the mother, noticeably aids any digestive discomfort of her baby. It is not a galactagogue, but if your little one has painful gas, constipation, or digestive issues, try drinking catnip tea – the benefits will pass through your milk. This made a huge difference for my little ones in their infancy. You can also give a weak catnip tea directly to your little one with a dropper.

Nourishing Herbs: Nourishing, vitamin & mineral rich herbs such as alfalfa, nettles, and raspberry leaf are helpful during breastfeeding for many reasons, including encouraging a plentiful milk supply.

Nourishing Foods: Eating nourishing foods, and as much of them as you want, is a key aspect of producing healthy, plentiful milk for your little one. Here are some foods that, in my experience, help to keep your milk supply plentiful: squash, dried (or fresh) apricots, figs (which also help the body to process and balance hormones,) sweet potatoes, and any starchy foods. White potatoes or Oatmeal are both incredibly effective at increasing milk in my personal experience, as is tapioca cooked in milk, with plenty of cream and egg yolk and maple syrup. Eating intuitively is key. Your body knows what it needs – listen to what it tells you. It is natural to gain weight during breastfeeding. Again, this is not a time to fast or restrict calories, since your milk supply will suffer.

Sleep: Getting enough sleep is probably the number one factor, in my experience, in producing plentiful milk. If your milk supply is low, take a look at your sleeping habits and adjust them if necessary. When my daughter was very young, she kept us up most of the night, and if I neglected to nap during the day, I wouldn't make enough milk. I know it can be hard to get enough sleep, especially during those first few months after birth. Listen to your body, and take every opportunity you can to rest if that is what your body needs.

Relaxation: Relaxation doesn't mean you need to sit around all day, unless that is what your body asks for. Relaxation means keeping stress to a minimum. Love yourself and carry out your daily life's work with ease and grace, and your milk supply will benefit. Certain herbs like oat straw, motherwort, and chamomile can be very helpful in promoting relaxation. Chamomile can be made into a tea, steeped only 10 minutes. Oat straw can be made into an infusion, and warm oatmeal has the same relaxing effect. Motherwort tincture can be used, 5 drops under the tongue or in water, every few hours if needed. Motherwort can cause dependency if used over a long period of time, so only use it in situations where you feel you would benefit, and not as a "preventative."

Herbs to Decrease Milk Supply

These herbs, along with some others not mentioned here, are known to decrease milk supply. They should be avoided while breastfeeding, unless you are attempting to wean your child or if you are experiencing very painful engorgement.

Sage: Sage is famously used to dry up milk supply, even when used in small amounts.

Parsley: I'll never forget the summer after my daughter was born, I was so excited when the flat-leaf Parsley we were growing had gotten big enough to start harvesting. I love Parsley! I put handfuls of it in all my food for a few days, and couldn't figure out why I wasn't making any milk! Then I learned that parsley has a reputation for drying up milk supply. A hot compress of parsley leaves on your breasts can also help to reduce milk supply, and relieve the pain associated with overfull breasts.

Herbs for Mastitis

The following herbs can be used to treat mastitis. (During the first few months of my daughter's life, I developed mastitis. At first I couldn't figure out why I was feeling terribly. Then I noticed I had a fever, and that my "blocked" milk duct had been blocked for a few days, and wasn't subsiding. I used echinacea, in tincture form, which helped clear the infection within a few hours.)

Echinacea: Susun Weed says she much prefers the action of echinacea infusion over the tincture, which is so widely used. She suggests 2 cups of infusion daily for mastitis, or ½ drop of tincture per pound of body weight up to 6 times a day. Continue use at lower dose for a day or two after the infection has cleared to ensure that it stays away.

Elder: Elder is immune strengthening, and an infusion of elder flowers is a good remedy for fever. Herbal lore tells us that the most potent elder medicine comes only from plants which one has developed an intimate relationship with. The Spirit of the plant must be willing to share her medicine for the gathered plant material to have any medicinal value. I believe this is true with any plant, but maybe it's more so with elder. Perhaps she is more discriminatory in regard to sharing her secrets & her healing powers.

Rose Hips & Vitamin C Rich Foods: Vitamin C helps to boost the immune system and helps your body heal from infection. Rose Hips contain a very high amount of vitamin C, well more than citrus fruits. Mix fresh powdered rose hips with just enough honey that it becomes stiff, like dough, but not particularly sticky. Roll this into balls about the size of a nickel and then roll them each in a bit of oat flour to make sure they don't get sticky – they can be sucked on liberally for a vitamin C boost.

Hot Compress, Comfrey Leaf & Marshmallow Root: Take a hot bath or shower or use a hot compress. Heat helps to sooth the breast tissue & fosters healing. Including herbs like comfrey leaf or marshmallow root in a hot compress helps to open clogged ducts & draws out the infection. Warmth and herbal compresses are also helpful in alleviating blocked milk ducts, even when mastitis is not a factor.

Sleep: Sleep deprivation is a major factor in the onset of mastitis. Lack of sleep lowers immune function & makes the body more vulnerable to infection. Getting enough sleep can facilitate the healing process. Sleep can also help to un-block milk ducts when mastitis is not a factor.

Postpartum Weight Gain

I seem to gain the most weight *after* the birth of my children, and not during pregnancy. Breastfeeding is a physically demanding job that requires a lot of energy, and so it is typical to be hungrier than usual during this time. According to Aviva Romm, a pregnant woman needs 2300 calories a day, while a nursing woman needs 2500. Breastfeeding women also need more of each vitamin and mineral (with the exception of Folic Acid which is needed more during pregnancy,) and need more carbohydrates (as opposed to protein, which is needed more during pregnancy.) This general need for more food-sourced nourishment as well as the fact that it's harder to move around with an infant in-arms often leads to postpartum weight gain. Postpartum weight gain is ok!

Cultural fear of being 'overweight' is quite real, and leads many women to try losing their 'baby weight' soon after giving birth. This can be detrimental, especially if the mother plans to breastfeed. During pregnancy a layer of fat is built for the sole purpose of being 'sucked back out' of you with your milk! Breastfeeding is more successful when the mother has a bit of cushioning.

Chances are that our partners will love our voluptuous postpartum bodies, and if they don't, that is something that can be discussed openly and with respect for the emotions on both sides.

Usually body weight returns to *your* normal within a few months to a few years of childbearing, but if not, maybe your body is really meant to be more voluptuous than it was pre-pregnancy. With each of my children, my body weight climbed steadily until around 7 months postpartum, and then naturally, slowly declined.

There are health implications for severe obesity, but there are even greater health implications for being severely underweight. Each of us has our own body type and our own optimally healthy weight. Instead of striving for a cultural ideal, we should strive for our own ideal by listening to our body and acting on our needs for rest, movement & nourishment.

Post-Partum Rest & Emotional Nurturing

"The moment a child is born, the mother is also born. She never existed before. The woman existed, but the mother, never. The mother is something absolutely new."

~*Osho*

The post-partum period is a time of powerful adjustment. The physical body is undergoing a rapid transformation from its pregnant to non-pregnant state. The baby is brand new to the world, learning in his own way what to expect and how to interact in this new environment. Hormones shift rapidly following birth, the mother's sleep patterns change, and her role as 'mother' is newborn too. She learns again how to walk, bathe, cook, sleep, communicate, nurture, and most importantly, she learns how to be nurtured.

A mother needs nurturing, care, and love just as does her newborn child. In traditional cultures, women understood this. The post-partum period usually included a time of rest – a period of time set aside for the mother and child to meet each other, to bond and communicate and nurture each other. Usually during this time, visitors would be minimized. The mothers, aunts, grandmothers and older sisters of the newborn mother, often the same women who attended the birth, would attend the post-partum period.

Different traditional cultures had, (and still have,) varying customs when it came to the post-natal period. The length of the mother's retreat with her newborn child varies, from only a few days, to a few weeks, to a full moon cycle or month, to a 40 day period, and in some cultures, two months or longer.

"Three months after the birth of her child, the Chagga woman's head is shaved and crowned with a bead tiara, she is robed in an ancient skin garment worked with beads, a staff such as the elders carry is put in her hand, and she

emerges from her hut for her first public appearance with her baby. Proceeding slowly towards the market, they are greeted with songs such as are sung to warriors returning from battle."

~ Carroll Dunham

There are usually differing components to this post-natal rest period, but there are four overlapping characteristics in almost all traditional cultures: warmth, massage, minimization of visitors, and a light or non-existent work-load. Some cultures also included medicinal herbs and plant remedies during this time. Some emphasized the importance of a diet consisting of only certain foods, and some included other practices, for instance, a custom called "belly-wrapping."

Warmth was by far considered the most important aspect of the post-partum period. A post-natal woman was brought warm soups, stews, and other warm foods to eat. She was brought warm water or herbal drinks, and discouraged from drinking cold water or eating any cold foods. Her living space was kept very warm, and she was often encouraged to perform certain rituals involving heat.

Malay communities in Malaysia & Indonesia incorporate two heat-related practices in their post-natal rest period. One practice involves a metal ball called a "Tuku," which is heated in the fire every morning, wrapped in cloth, and rolled gently over the woman's abdomen. The second ritual involves a wooden apparatus called a "Salai," which is positioned a foot or two over a bed of hot coals. The woman lies on the wooden bed each afternoon, letting the warmth from the coals penetrate and relax her whole body. The Malay post-natal period lasts 40 to 48 days, and these heat-related practices are part of a group of daily rituals including full-body massage, belly wrapping, herbal tonics, and a special diet.

"Regardless of the tribe, the use of heat had four main purposes: to prevent excessive bleeding; to bring down the mother's milk; to offer her post-birth comfort; and to help shrink the uterus."

~Veronika Sophia Robinson

Massage, another traditional post-partum ritual, has immeasurable benefits for new mothers. Massage improves circulation, helps ease cramps and muscle aches, helps the body process hormones, relaxes the body & the mind, and soothes the emotions. Many cultures massaged the belly soon after birth, to aid in the expulsion of the placenta, and continued with gentle daily belly massages after birth to ensure swift & proper uterine involution, (return of the uterus to the normal pre-pregnancy size.) Most cultures, however, did not just focus on the belly – post-partum massage was usually a lengthy & relaxing full body massage with countless benefits to the new mother.

In Malay communities, the ritual of post-partum massage is called Mengurut Badan. In some modern Malay families, professional massage therapists, trained in post-partum massage, visit the new mother for 45 minutes to an hour every day during the 40 day post-partum period.

In parts of Southern India, where the post-partum rest period sometimes lasts as long as 60 days, women are traditionally given a full body massage, called a 'maalish,' every day during that period. Women in most traditional African, European, Asian and American Indian cultures received post-partum massage daily from their mothers, midwives, grandmothers, or older female family members. This practice continued for many weeks after the birth.

The workload of new mothers, across the board in traditional cultures, was lightened by their family and tribe. Women were not expected to cook or care for younger children, clean, or carry out any strenuous chores. Women were usually especially discouraged from heavy lifting.

Belly wrapping, practiced in many traditional cultures, was believed to help the uterus return to its pre-pregnancy size, and to help the abdominal muscles and internal organs regain their pre-pregnancy placement in the belly. Most cultures used a long wide piece of cloth or animal hide for this purpose. In Malay culture, this belly wrap is called 'barut.' It is tightly wrapped around the abdomen, and usually worn through the night, taken off in the morning, worn again during the mid-day, and then taken off again in the afternoon for the entire 40-48 day post-partum rest period.

Often during pregnancy, modern women are told observer accounts of traditional women giving birth in the fields, slinging their newborn baby onto their back, and resuming work immediately. While this may be true, my feeling is that these women probably had no other choice. Poverty and scarcity necessitate many practices that are less than ideal for optimal health and well-being. Women who were able to engage in a post-partum rest period usually did so.

Many modern women refer to this post-partum sabbatical as a 'babymoon.' Modern women who engage in a babymoon usually try to engage in many of the traditional practices mentioned above, keeping visitors to a minimum and resting as much as possible for a certain amount of time. This time-frame depends on the mother's personal preference and ability to receive help, but a babymoon usually lasts anywhere from a few days to a few weeks.

Unfortunately, many modern women do not have the support necessary to foster any post-partum rest period. The tribal family model has been replaced in many cases with a nuclear family model, and in many cases, with the single parent model. New mothers without support are forced to resume work right away; they are forced to cook and clean and to care for toddlers or older children in the immediate post-partum period. This lack of support can quickly lead to post-partum depression and complete exhaustion.

The maternity care system in the United States is bleak and suboptimal. With so much emphasis on pregnancy and birth care, it is surprising to me that after the birth, many women are left with absolutely no support.

*"Is ours not a strange culture that focuses so much attention
on childbirth — virtually all of it based on anxiety and fear
— and so little on the crucial time after birth, when patterns
are established that will affect the individual and the family
for decades?"*

~Suzanne Arms

Whenever possible, find post-partum support. In many U.S. cities, there are women's groups dedicated to free post-partum maternal care. If this is not the case near you, many student doulas will work for free in exchange for experience gained. Partners, family members and friends should all understand that their support would be welcomed and much appreciated. Even an hour a week, if that is all that is possible, can make all the difference.

*"When you study postpartum depression, there is a very
clear understanding that in communities where you see more
support, there is less depression."*

~Ariel Gore

Post-partum rest and rehabilitation is not only incredibly beneficial to the new mother, but also to her infant. A relaxed, well rested and emotionally stable mother is better suited to care for and nourish her infant. Sleep deprivation and stress are the main causes of an insufficient milk supply. This period is essential for mother-child bonding, and provides an opportunity for the baby to become acquainted with his surroundings, gently and lovingly.

If no external support is possible during the post-partum period, new mothers can and do learn to support themselves. This self-support, given the right circumstances, can offer good health, strength, and emotional wellbeing. Svea Boyda-Vikander, in her article Mothering the New Mother, puts it very clearly: "While 40 days of rest is not realistic to those of us who need to look after other children, go to school, or work to pay bills, we can change our attitudes about what is expected of ourselves and other women post-partum."

Holding to this post-partum period of rest is not about superstition, although it has taken that form in many cultures. It is not about mandated bed-rest or mandated sexual abstinence. It is not about limiting spicy foods, if spicy is what you crave, or about binding your abdomen if it feels uncomfortable to you. This post-partum period, as with any other period in the childbearing cycle, is most healing and nourishing if you are able to hear your inner voice and follow your intuition. If your body desires a walk outdoors with your newborn, do not confine yourself to a house because it is tradition. If you feel like a cold glass of milk is really what your body desires, then don't restrict yourself to only warm foods because that is a standard of post-partum care. This period is really about rest – not bed rest, but true rest. It is not about following the paths of your ancestors, but about following the path of your heart. It is about connecting with your newborn, and learning together the true meaning of nourishment.

> "As a culture, we have woefully neglected the needs of new mothers. But this was not always so. Historically, we recognized the importance of a community of women helping women, who provided this much needed practical and emotional assistance. In so doing, they provided a chance for postpartum women to recuperate and assimilate the major change that had taken place in their lives…. Women can make a comfortable and peaceful transition into motherhood. Postpartum mental illness is not inevitable and in many cases can be prevented. It is time that we recognize and meet the needs of postpartum women. The health of our families depends on it."
>
> ~Kathleen Kendall-Tackett

Post-Partum Ceremony & Ritual

*"In cultures were a strong tradition of ritual or ceremony is
honored and regularly practiced, there is an emphasis on
being in the world, rather than doing tasks or accomplishing
things… an emphasis on the process of deepening, rather
than the process of producing and achieving…. Earth-
honoring peoples from cultures around the world, ancient
times to the present, use ceremony to sustain the health and
cohesiveness of individuals and community. There is much to
learn from these peoples and their ways, for they speak
clearly of humans' true spiritual essence and of our deep
connection to Mother Earth."*

~Gail Faith Edwards

The birth of a child is a sacred event. In traditional cultures it was
viewed as such, and sacred rituals surrounding birth were practiced.
In many cultures, the placenta, the caul, and the umbilical cord held a
very special place in those rituals, as did the name given to the child,
the entrance of the child into his or her tribe, and the initiation of the
mother into the community of motherhood.

Rituals surrounding the placenta, caul, and umbilical cord often
served the purpose of connecting the infant with her tribe's ancestral
land. Placental rituals in traditional cultures also served to protect the
mother and child, to ensure that the child would not wander as an
adult, and to respect the sacred relationship between the child and
the placenta.

*"When the cord falls off, it is understood that the newborn
now not only belongs to the mother, but to the whole
community. Traditionally an animal is slaughtered as a
sacrifice and the skin of the animal is given to the new
infant as a protective clothing or sleeping mat. The burial*

spot of the placenta seals the attachment of a person to their ancestral land and it is a place to which many will return as adults. This burial place of the placenta is a place to connect with their ancestors in times of trouble, to dream and eventually to die."

~ Marianne Littlejohn on traditional Khoisan birth rituals in South Africa

In many cultures, the placenta would be buried in a place that held special significance to the mother, and in some agrarian societies, a special tree would be planted over the placenta.

Traditional naming ceremonies had many intentions. They served to initiate a child into the tribe, or to connect the infant with a certain ancestor. Often times, infants would carry the name of a relative, then deceased, whose gifts and talents brought joy or prosperity to the tribe. In other cultures, infants would be given a brand new name, and the name was thought to solidify their path in life. Sobonfu Some describes a ritual from her tribe, the Dagara of Africa, called the 'hearing ritual.' In this ritual, a group of elders convenes with the mother during her pregnancy. She is put into a trance-like state, and the elders speak to the child within, asking the child why she has come. The child speaks using the mother's voice, and the elders design a name to fit the child's purpose in life. The mother is brought back, and the elders hold the name until the child is born. The name is then given to the child a few days after the birth. 'Sobonfu' means keeper of the ritual. She now travels, speaking and writing about the rituals of her tribe and the importance of ritual for our health as a species, in the hopes of bringing ritual back to others in the modern world.

In other cultures, specifically in some Native American tribes, babies were not given names until much later in life, or were given different names at different points in life. As an infant, the baby would be called "little one." Their names would be given, in time, as emblems of their growing spirit and direction.

Another moment which holds special significance in many cultures, and which is often ritualized, it the end of the post-partum rest period, where the mother and the newborn rejoin their tribe. In some cases, this moment is the first meeting of the newborn baby with her father, as in almost all cultures men were not allowed to attend birth. The mother and newborn were often bathed and given new or special garments to wear upon their re-entrance into the tribe.

Integrating ritual and ceremony into our own birth journeys does not necessarily mean reproducing what our ancestors did. Personally, placental burial rituals and conscious naming ceremonies resonate with me, but ceremony is personal, and does not need to follow a certain structure. Ceremony can take infinite forms – ceremony is about deepening our connection to ourselves, to our children, to the earth, and to the spiritual nature of life.

Healing Herbs for the Postpartum Period

Comfrey – All parts of the comfrey plant have amazing healing properties. Comfrey's Latin name, Symphytum, literally means "to bring together." Its healing properties can be absorbed through the skin, making it an excellent herb to use as a poultice. It is also incredibly healing when used as an infusion, or as a tincture.

During the post-partum period, comfrey can be helpful in many ways. Comfrey poultices can be helpful for healing tears or trauma to the vagina, or for soothing sore nipples during breastfeeding. To make a poultice, wrap a handful of fresh or dried comfrey leaves in a clean cotton cloth, and tie it with a string. Put the wrapped comfrey leaves into a small jar (just big enough for the wrapped leaved to fit comfortably) and pour boiling water over them, just as you would when making a regular infusion. Let the comfrey steep until the water has cooled slightly. The water should still be quite warm. Take the wrapped comfrey out and apply them, cloth and all, to the part of you that needs healing: vagina, breasts, wherever. You can continue to poultice with the remaining liquid in the jar. (You can also make a poultice using the bruised fresh (mature) leaves, whole and unwrapped, but they can be scratchy and irritating when used this way.)

Comfrey leaf infusion, one cup a day for a week or two, can have amazing healing benefits and can begin to quickly alleviate the pain of perennial tears. This can also speed the postpartum recovery process in general.

Comfrey can also be added to baths to promote healing. This could take the form of a conventional bath, or a small sitz bath in a basin, just big enough to sit in.

In recent years, comfrey has come under some scrutiny. Comfrey contains alkaloids which could be damaging to the liver. According to Gail Faith Edwards, however, a cup of red wine has 144 times more 'harmful' alkaloids than one cup of comfrey leaf infusion. To top that, most of the alkaloids are concentrated in the young leaves and roots, and not in the mature leaves. In my opinion, isolating a compound and saying a plant is dangerous because of one of its infinite components does not make sense. Plants work best in their whole form. Comfrey has an age old tradition in the world of healing plants, which I believe speaks to its safety.

Comfrey is the one and only herb that I actively sought out during my second pregnancy because of its innumerable post-partum benefits. It often grows in old fields, near barns and old farmhouses. Once comfrey is established, it is hard to "uproot." Each broken root piece, however small, yields a new plant. Perhaps this is a symbol of its healing capacity: from what is broken, fractured, torn or severed, comfrey will aid in new and vibrant growth, without fail.

Comfrey is also a beneficial herb for the heart, making it an even more beautiful herb for postpartum mothers. If you harvest comfrey yourself, always harvest the mature leaves, from the Comfrey plants with purple, not white, flowers.

Dandelion – Dandelion, leaf and root, is not in any way specific to the postpartum period. Rather, it is a tonic for general health, strengthening to the whole body, and seems like it deserves a place in this list.

Dandelion is an aid to the liver. When the liver is functioning optimally, the body is able to more easily process the hormones of birth and the postpartum period. Dandelion is also a digestive aid and a very, very mild diuretic. It strengthens the heart, which is an invaluable asset to a new mother, and is an excellent overall tonic for the urinary and reproductive systems as well as the immune & lymphatic systems.

Drink a cup or two of dandelion root infusion every few days during the postpartum period, or use 30 drops of tincture every few days.

Catnip –Catnip tea is relaxing, eases cramps, and can aid in lessening the pain of uterine contractions which continue for a few days after birth, known as afterpains.

Catnip is also a digestive aid for both the mother and newborn. If your baby has digestive discomfort, painful gas, or constipation, the digestive benefits of catnip will pass through your milk to him, helping to relax his intestines and ease digestion.

You can drink catnip tea as often as you wish throughout the postpartum period. After the births of my first two children, I added it to teas and infusions. The longer it steeps, the more bitter it tastes.

Susun Weed also suggests that if you need immediate relief, catnip can be smoked.

Ground Ivy – Susun Weed suggests Ground Ivy for afterpains and to "promote good uterine tone."

Nettle – Nettle leaf is a beautiful tonic herb to use after birth. It helps to tone the genito-urinary system and can provide relief from fatigue and exhaustion. Nettle also contain high stores of iron, an essential mineral during the postpartum period, and can increase milk flow.

I suggest drinking a cup of nettle infusion a day, during the entire postpartum period and beyond, to impart overall health and vitality.

Echinacea – Echinacea is also a helpful herb to have around during the postpartum period. Echinacea boosts the immune system, and be helpful in any cases of maternal infections, including mastitis or childbed fever.If the newborn develops an infection, Echinacea will pass through the mother's milk to her infant.

Motherwort – Motherwort is my favorite herb for the postpartum period, and for the journey of motherhood as a whole. Motherwort strengthens the heart – It imparts courage and poise in times of stress, and provides a calm and centered presence in times of overwhelm.

Motherwort is also an amazing tonic for the uterus. It can support swift healing in the postpartum period, and at the same time is one of the herbs most often used to relieve the pain of postpartum uterine contractions.

Unlike many other nervous-system tonics, motherwort does not cause sleepiness, but rather a peacefully and attentively centered presence.

Motherwort increases circulation and brings warmth to the body, which, as many traditional cultures knew, is a necessary aspect of healing during the postpartum period. Motherwort is also one of the best herbs to use, supplemented with self-nourishment and self-love, in the treatment of postpartum depression and anxiety disorders.

Gail Faith Edwards writes that through her observation, "motherwort not only supports us emotionally, but also teaches, through her growing habit and appearance, a lesson for strong emotional health. The prickly parts of our natures, the parts we usually try to hide and stuff away, need to be acknowledged and allowed to coexist with our softer, more socially acceptable parts. Motherwort encourages us to embrace and nourish those hard parts of ourselves."

Some women, like me, feel five drops of Motherwort tincture acting quickly to calm and center. Others may need double or triple that dose to notice the effects. Motherwort comes with a mild caution: Do not use motherwort in lieu of self-nurturing. Dependencies can be formed, and motherwort should not be used for more than a few weeks at a time, unless the use is sporadic. Instead, look to your own healing capacity – avoid stress – rest often – love your body – eat well – nourish your spirit... and if, in the course of this self-care, stress and emotional fatigue materialize, as they sometimes do along the path of motherhood, then call on Motherwort as your ally.

A Recipe for Baby Balm:

1 part fresh wilted Calendula flowers

1 Part fresh wilted Rose Petals

1 Part fresh wilted Chamomile Flowers

Olive Oil

Beeswax

Directions: Place flowers into a glass jar. Cover with olive oil. Make sure there are no air bubbles. Place the jar in on very warm windowsill or in another warm place, like on a shelf above a woodstove, for one week. The ideal temperature for the oil to infuse is 90 to 100 degrees. Strain the oil into another jar with cheesecloth, and squeeze remaining oil from the herbs gently. You can also infuse in a double boiler or a warm oven for a few hours for a similar effect.

Melt 1 oz. beeswax in a glass or metal salve container using a double boiler. Add 4 oz. of flower-infused olive oil, once the beeswax has melted. Let the mixture melt again, remove from heat, and stir well. Let cool.

This balm is amazing in treating diaper rash and chapped skin. It is gentle enough for newborn babies, but can also be used to soothe sore nipples or as a general purpose healing balm.

Part V:

Three Freebirth Stories

"When you walk to the edge of all the light you have

and take that first step into the darkness of the unknown,

you must believe that one of two things will happen:

There will be something solid for you to stand upon,

or, you will be taught how to fly."

~Patrick Overton

Peacy's Story

March 10, 2011

It's the middle of the night. I'mlying awake, thinking of how there will be three of us sleeping here soon. I can't lay still. I'm feeling different, off, restless - Every once in a while, I'm compelled to get up on all fours and rock back and forth. I don't think a whole lot of it - I'm not expecting Peacy to come for another week, even two. It doesn't occur to me yet that this might be the beginnings of labor!

A Bit of Background

In late February of 2011, Joey and I drove from Maine to New Hampshire to move into our new house, a tiny log cabin with no running water or electricity. I was about eight & a half months pregnant. The snow was so deep that winter; we had to bring all our belongings down to the cabin by way of a sled. I spent our first week there sewing curtains for the windows & making sheets for our new bed. It was so cozy and warm there - I felt safe and comfortable, and so relieved to be moved from our dark, cold house in Maine.

Peacy was born about a week after moving to our new home.

March 10, Around Midnight

Sleep isn't coming. Something tells me to use the potty. Maybe this is all it is - I just need to go poop and then I'll be able to sleep. The outhouse is a minutes' walk from our cabin, and although it's March, it's still very surely winter. But, I have to poop - what else am I going to do? I throw on a big flannel shirt, climb down the ladder, and head outside. I make my way through the snow, huddled against the chill wind. There's a bit of an icy path to follow, but its dark, and every once in a while I step off the path and find myself knee-deep in the snow. I make it to the outhouse, sit on the potty, and go poop. Then I make my way back to the cabin and open the door to find the warm relief of the woodstove. Ahhh, I can relax! I crawl back into bed next to Joey.

Still no sleep. I have to poop again. Not again! I just got warm! Flannel shirt back on. Out the door, to the outhouse...

After a few trips outside in the freezing wind, I decide to give up on sleeping. I light a candle, (our only source of light at night save the moon,) and stay downstairs near the woodstove. There is obviously something going on now. I'm hot one minute & and then I've got chills the next, and I can't sit still. I begin to suspect, just maybe, that my little girl is on her way.

Then I really notice the contractions – they are pretty close together, maybe once every 3 minutes. They're short and mild, very bearable, but growing in intensity.

Suddenly, I'm very cold. The fire in the woodstove has died down – there are only a few embers left. I attempt to make another fire. Usually, I consider myself a pretty skilled fire-maker. I start to break up the slightly soggy kindling as best I can, (jumping on it between contractions.) I squat down, and what I've managed to break to a decently small size I pile into the woodstove. I light a bit of birch bark to get the fire going, and the flames start to rise, and then a contraction comes!

The contractions are getting stronger, and require much more energy. My attention is pulled away from the woodstove into my pelvis. I close my eyes & rock back & forth, immersing myself in the rush of energy. When the contraction passes, I look up to see a whole lot of smoke, but no flames. This goes on for a while. Every time I try to light the fire, another contraction comes! Soon, there's a charred, smoking mass of kindling in the fire, and there I am, cold & bouncing around in front of the woodstove. Finally, my ridiculously persistent drive to do things myself gives in to the reality of the situation. I call upstairs to Joey.

Joey comes down the ladder, groggy, and comments on the smoking mass of kindling that was my attempted fire. I smile and relax. He starts a blazing fire in a matter of minutes. I tell him I think Peacy is coming. The cabin begins to warm up, the fire in the stove roaring and red hot, and my contractions get much stronger. I spend most of my time on my knees, my torso resting on the edge of the couch, swaying and moaning, and then resting when they pass. Joey rubs my back and brings me water. I can tell he is tired. I'm tired too. In between contractions, I lay down on the couch with him. A few times, I try to let the contractions come while laying down, but it's too intense, almost unbearable, and each time I end up back on my knees, bent over the couch, moaning my earth chant & pulling all my power into my pelvis to speed my baby's passage.

I need to rest – It's only been a few hours since I noticed the beginnings of labor, but the contractions are so strong and relentless… I am so tired. Finally, rest comes. Joey and I drift off to sleep, laying together on the couch, in the pre-dawn darkness.

March 10, Just After Sunrise

I wake up to the most brilliant light! Our little cabin is illuminated by the sunlight beaming through the windows, spilling over onto the walls and the ceiling and the couch where we still lay. It is so beautiful and breathtaking! Contractions start again right away, as fast and intense as they had been before we fell asleep. Joey starts to steep some herbs for me to drink after the birth. The contractions are so strong now that I can't even get up to get myself water, or even to go pee!

I'm on my hands and knees – the only position that feels comfortable – rocking and moaning through the contractions which seem to be coming every minute. Joey brings me water when all I can manage to say is "water," and he brings me containers to go pee into when I need to.

He rubs my back, I think maybe because he's not quite sure what else to do to support me. During an especially intense contraction, he rubs my back again. "Don't do that!" He stops. I need every ounce of my attention. Even a back rub is too much for me to handle, too distracting. Sometimes there is pain, although not unbearable. I rock my way through it. My moans are louder, filled with tension – sometimes they are grunts, even screams.

About an hour after sunrise, I feel a swelling in the birth canal. This is such a powerful moment – I can really feel her – she is so close! Somehow, through all those months of her growing inside of me, it never really hit me that she was real – now it hits me! The contractions are so intense that I don't even really feel them, (or at least that is what my memory tells me!) I am in the most beautiful trance – I can feel her so close!!

Soon, I feel her pushing against the wall of my vagina – her door to the world. I put my hand back to feel her. So incredible! I can feel her! But… is that her? It doesn't feel like a head! I ask Joey to look. He agrees - it doesn't look like a head, or like any part of a baby. It looks like a membrane. Then I realize my waters never broke! It's the caul! She keeps going back up inside me and then pushing back down. I can feel her with my hand, and I feel like I'm stretching as much as I can. I even try pushing her out, but she's not even close to crowning.

I ask Joey to look in our copy of "Spiritual Midwifery" to see if he can find anything about what's happening. I want to know if it's ok for us to break the caul, or if I should just keep trying with the caul intact. Joey reads for a bit, while Peacy keeps going in and out. He finds something on late rupture of membranes, but nothing helpful. I ask him to break the caul – he uses his fingernail and breaks it. Relief! Instantly I feel freer, and can tell that Peacy does too. Her head starts to crown!

Peacy crowns for a minute. I let out a grunt-scream-bellow-cry, and my body gives an enormous involuntary push, followed by a very voluntary, very strained push, and her head is out!! Her body follows easily, along with a rush of waters and a bit of blood. Joey catches her and holds her as I turn to take her. I hold her to my breast.

Peacy is blue and wailing, and quickly turns pink. She is pudgy and squat and round and so perfect! I have never seen such a perfect, beautiful being! Our dog Naya, who I had forgotten about completely, comes running over to sniff this strange, loud, new little thing. I'm afraid Naya is going to bite Peacy, or eat her! I tell Joey to put Naya outside, which he does.

Peacy definitely does not want to nurse! She cries and squirms and cries some more. I cry with joy. She is so beautiful, so so so beautiful! I could never have imagined!!! The light in Joey's eyes is so bright and beautiful as he looks at her.

My body feels so strange. My belly is limp and squishy.

The placenta comes. Joey ties Peacy's cord and cuts it. I eat a tiny bite of the placenta, (not exactly my idea of tasty, but it certainly feels nourishing,) and then Joey wraps it in a towel and places it in a cupboard, (where I proceed to forget about it until a few days later.)

Joey holds Peacy for a long time. She sleeps in his arms while I clean myself and the cabin up. Naya is outside, scratching at the door to come back in – she is so curious. We let her in, finally. I try going pee outside in the snow. It burns – stings – it is so painful. I have a tear, in the front, right by my pee-hole, probably because of that last strained push as her head came through.

I don't remember when it was, during all this, that she opened her eyes for the first time, but I remember being completely blown away.

Her eyes were the deepest blue I had ever seen. They were infinite, profound, and deep as the furthest reaches of space and the deepest depths of the ocean.

March 10 -15, 2011

The next few days were a struggle. Peacy didn't seem to want to eat or sleep, so we didn't get to eat or sleep much either. I remember being so exhausted one night that I passed out right next to Peacy while she was wailing. Finally she took to nursing. There were a lot of diapers to wash and dry – we got water from the stream and heated it on the woodstove to wash the diapers in, and strung the clean, wet diapers above the woodstove to dry. Joey did pretty much everything for me those first few days – it was a good lesson for me in accepting help. He made me amazing soups and went out to do food shopping; he walked up the hill to collect our drinking water and washed all the diapers. Although it was challenging, I'll never forget those first few days. They were so beautiful.

I remember the first time we took Peacy outside, a few days after she was born, all bundled up in a million blankets, and we walked through the snow with her to the Maple Sugar Shack to talk with Steve, the man who was renting the cabin to us. We walked into the shack, greeted by the smell of boiling maple sap and a look of surprise on Steve's face. "You had your baby!" And then, "Aren't you supposed to put up a flag or something?!" It was so good to feel the lightheartedness of Steve's presence. Something about his words brought me back to reality a little. They felt like a testament to what a monumental undertaking this all was – and, to the fact that this was something all mothers and fathers do – something Steve had done three times! It felt like a consecration – a blessing from Steve in his own way.

April, 2011

Peacy's name took a long time to come. At first I called her little-one, and that was perfect. We called her Squirmo, because she was never still except when she slept, and all sorts of other names for fun, but her full name did not come.

Before Peacy's birth, Joey had told me of a Native American tradition where children's names were constantly in motion – constantly changing based on their phase of life and their spirit. I tried this out with Peacy, but it didn't feel right; I wanted her to have a name of her own – it felt like something she was entitled to, something sacred. I thought about it for a long time... I over-thought it. I came up with a name, Lynnea, and I shared it with Joey. He didn't like it. He asked me why I had chosen it. I told him it reminded me of the forsythia – the first vibrant blossom of the spring.

"What about 'Spring Blossom,'" he said.

I fell in love with this – I had never even considered a name so beautiful – Over the next few months, her name evolved. It became like a poem. It came to embody her soft, radiant beauty, her fiery spirit, and her deeply passionate soul. We gave her a nickname too, "Peacy," because who can say "Apple Blossom Light Hawk Summer Willow Wind, come get your dinner!!"

Micah's Story

Micah was conceived a few days after Peacy's first birthday. It was a beautiful night – a crescent moon hanging, white and luminous, above the tall pine trees that grew to the west of our little cabin. Venus and Jupiter twinkling, side by side on the horizon, in that magical half-light just after sunset… the first night of Micah's journey inside of me. So, there were to be two!

About a month in to my pregnancy, I could tell he was a boy. I could feel his spirit was much calmer and quieter than his sister's, like he was always watching and waiting, taking his time.

I knew well from the beginning that Micah's birth would be a freebirth too. I had so much confidence in my body, and my friends and family were all much more accepting and supportive of the choice this time around.

Micah's birth started very much like Peacy's, except by then we had moved to a different town in Maine, where we had found another family to live with. We had just finished building a cabin on their land that would be our sleeping cabin, and we shared the main house for cooking, washing, bathing & meals.

We had spent part of the summer and fall camping on that land, while Joey worked on building the cabin. When we finally moved into our little sleeping cabin in November, it was so revitalizing. We had a warm place to sleep and a comfortable bed; a place to settle down, relax, and have a bit more privacy.

I spent the weeks just before Micah's birth sewing curtains for our cabin's windows.

I was so ready to meet this calm, beautiful little boy!

December 8, 2012, the night of Micah's Birth:

I am irritable. I'm emotionally volatile. I want to be alone. We're in the main house trying to get dinner ready for our two families, and it's hard to find the time and the space for privacy. I can't stand all the commotion. I end up crouching down behind the stove, where there's a little secluded space under a shelf. I take a deep breath. I don't know why I'm so irritable!

After dinner Joey & I take Peacy out to our sleeping cabin. It's dark and quiet and I feel relaxed again. There's just enough space for our huge family bed (a queen mattress pushed up next to a twin,) in the bigger room of the cabin. I'm so grateful for the soft candlelight. Peacy, who's about 21 months old now, has trouble going to sleep as usual, but finally lays still and eventually closes her eyes. Joey and I lay down next to one another, but after a few minutes, I don't feel ready for sleep, and I go back to the main house.

John and Nyla, (who are sharing the main house & land with us) are inside sweeping and doing the dishes from dinner. Their two little boys, 5 years old and 7 months old, are there too. I offer to help clean up but they have done most of the work already, and seem happy to finish. Grateful for the opportunity, I go into the bathroom and start to fill a warm bath.

The water is so relaxing. I feel like maybe it will help me sleep well tonight. After the bath I wrap myself in a towel and walk the snowy little pathway back out to our sleeping cabin. It's so warm, dark, and quiet. Peacy and Joey are both asleep. I lay down with them and drift in and out of peaceful dreams.

December 8, 11PM

I wake up needing to go poop. We have a sawdust composting toilet next to the woodstove in our tiny entryway room; we call it the "potty bucket." After I use the potty bucket, I have trouble going back to sleep... I feel restless... I recognize this feeling! I'm not expecting Micah to come for another two weeks, but I suspect that these feelings are very mild contractions!

My body wants the soothing warmth of the bath again. I climb into bed with Joey to tell him that I think Micah is on his way, and that I'm going back to the bath. I tell him I'll come back if it feels right, but somehow I know I won't. I know Micah will be born in the main house.

All the lights are still on when I walk in the door to the main house, and John and Nyla are still up, talking. I'm surprised they're still awake! The lights feel blinding – they hurt my eyes. I stop in the doorway, looking at them. I was not expecting to meet anyone – I feel like a deer in headlights! A light contraction comes and then passes. Nyla asks me what's going on. I start to explain, feeling guilty about taking two baths in one night. I'm holding my belly, moving it around a bit because it seems to ease the feelings. Nyla very clearly knows what's going on. As I'm rambling about the bath, a stronger contraction comes. Micah is telling me to shut up and get in the bath! I comply, thankful to let go of my guilt about using too much hot water.

I light a candle and turn off the lights in the bathroom. I'm relaxed again, back in a dimly lit and comfortable space. The hot water feels so amazing. The contractions get a little stronger. I no longer feel remotely sleepy – there is a powerful energy running through me, like waves of light. At first, I sit still in the bath, but that doesn't last long. I move into all sorts of positions. The bathtub feels restrictively small – I can't find my ideal position, but the water is so nice. I jiggle my belly with my hands when the contractions come, and sing a low, almost inaudibly low note – my earth chant again, but more refined this time. I keep thinking maybe this isn't labor after all, it is so mild. I feel so calm and spacious and steady.

Nyla knocks on the door and asks me if I need anything. I ask her for tea. She brings it to me, and brings me some towels to drape over the hard edges of the bath. Both the tea and the towels are a great comfort. She sits with me for a while. "I keep thinking this isn't labor," I say. She just smiles. Of course it is labor! She breathes with me and tells me I am beautiful. At one point, I need to go poop and feel a little embarrassed for a moment. Then I let that go. My body needs me to let go. I get out of the bath to use the potty bucket.

John leaves the main house to go out to his and Nyla's cabin, where their two boys are sleeping. All the lights in the main house are off now. Then, in the bathroom, we hear the sound of their younger boy's beautiful little voice coming through the baby monitor. We hear him wake up, and then start to cry. Nyla gets up to go out to him; she seems conflicted for a moment, unsure if I want her to stay with me. My body is glad at the idea of being alone. I ask her not come back. "How will I know if you need anything?"

"I'll turn the house lights on if I need any help."

December 8, Midnight

Things speed up so quickly! I hadn't realized how much inhibition I had been feeling. Now I am alone – I feel completely safe and unreserved – I really am able to let go, and it is so, so, so powerful!!! It is a beautiful blur! Contractions are coming one after another, and so strong. I realize the bathroom is not where I want to be.

I leave the bath and head out into the rest of the house. There is a candle burning – it is luminous, swirling. The whole house seems to swirl around me. I am rocked by such a powerful contraction as I am walking, and it brings me to my knees. It is mind-blowing. I don't feel in control of my body – it seems to have an intelligence so far beyond my mind! Micah is coming so quickly!!!

I want access to the potty bucket. I feel like I have to go pee, but I don't want to be in the bathroom. I feel super-human! Somehow, I manage to drag the whole potty bucket contraption and a bunch of towels out of the bathroom and into the kitchen/living room through those infinitely powerful contractions! For some reason, I want to be right there by the couch. It feels so right. My body does this before I even have a second to think about it. I sit on the potty to go pee, but I jump up almost immediately, almost involuntarily, and then fall to the floor on my hands and knees. I feel him!! He is right there in the birth canal, so close!!

I smile with such joy!! I don't remember ever in my life feeling so much joy and pure elation! I say his name, (for this time around, I know his name.) It feels like pure light flowing from my mouth as I say it, almost out of breath: "Micah Starlight Rowan Flower Frost!!!" My whole being is pure, blissful love. I say his name again, and there is another burst of infinite love! How can this get any more beautiful?!!!! I call him again and again and again!

"Micah Starlight Rowan Flower Frost! Micah Starlight Rowan Flower Frost!!!"

And then, so quickly, Micah is right there, swelling, opening me. With my hand, reaching back underneath me, I feel his head start to crown. I feel the caul is still over his head but there is no time to think about if I should break it this time. He goes back inside me for just a moment and then crowns again. I hold his head as he pushes through. There is no way to describe the intensity of the love in this moment. I catch him as he slides out, and bring him forward all in one motion. The caul falls away and reveals his body, waters spilling to the floor. He so tiny and blue, choking and sputtering. I feel the cord is around his neck. I struggle with it for a moment, recklessly trying to pull him free, but then he does a little flip in my hands and unwinds it himself!

Micah breathes. I hold him to my chest, stand up, and walk to the bathroom, followed by a trail of little drops of blood on the floor. I get into the bath and the water immediately turns red. I gaze at him.

His eyes are open, slate-blue like the ocean on a quiet, cloudy day.

He is looking around. I suddenly feel very cold. I feel like I need help. I turn on the bathroom light, and he starts to cry, but I talk to him, sooth him. He looks up at me, so innocent and beautiful and trusting. He is so small, the smallest baby I have ever seen. (We never weigh him, but later on when he's about a week old, we compare him to a 5 lb. bag of apples and figure he weighs about the same.)

December 9, From Midnight to Sunrise:

Joey and Nyla make a big fire in the woodstove and push a comfortable chair up next to the warmth. I sit in the chair, and Micah nurses right away. The placenta comes. There is a lot of blood – more than there ever was with Peacy's birth. I feel what I think is a huge clot, or a part of the placenta that didn't make its way out, right at the opening of my vagina in the back. It doesn't hurt so I try to loosen it, but it's clearly attached. (A day later, the midwife who attended Nyla's younger son's birth comes to check me – it turns out it is a rather bad tear where the blood is pooling and clotting. She says I'm very lucky it doesn't hurt.)

Joey ties and cuts Micah's cord. He and Nyla help me onto the couch, which they've pushed up near the woodstove – I'll sleep on the couch tonight; making my way out to our sleeping cabin seems like too much right now. I just want to hold this sweet little boy. He fits right on my shoulder, he is so small. Nyla makes me some cereal with blueberries and molasses, and she and Joey both go back to sleep.

I lay there in the main house, drifting in and out of a very light sleep. Micah sleeps so well, and wakes to nurse often. I watch the moon rise just before dawn – it is a luminous sliver, just as it was on the night he was conceived. Then I watch the sky turn pink, and then gold, and then see the sun come up. It illuminates the house, quietly beaming through the windows onto the wood floor. Micah's first sunrise.

Out in our cabin, Peacy wakes up. Joey gets her dressed and brings her into the main house, to meet her new little brother. She is interested, slightly, but she's more interested in having breakfast.

Ahmik's Story

Your beginning ~ spring, 2015

I was out planting potatoes the day after Beltane – a few days before the May full moon. I had expected my period to come a few days earlier, but there was still no sign.

After moving to a little village in New Mexico the previous fall, we had finally gotten our chickens, and some rabbits too… the rabbits had already had babies. We were in the process of reclaiming a beautiful old garden by the house from the wild mustard and crab-grass. Little carrots, lettuces and parsley were already sprouting. We were putting the finishing touches on the small goat barn we were building, expecting to pick up 5 baby goats in a few weeks.

That spring was a busy one. Some sort of wildfire had been ignited within me, and after years of up-rootedness, moving again and again from one house to the next, I was determined to make this one my home – resolute in my ambition to finally set down some roots! That spring I was in building mode, planning mode, gardening mode – having another baby was really the last thing on my mind!

But the May full moon came and went, and still no period. I began to suspect that you were there, a tiny seed sprouting in the garden of my womb. You came to me so quietly that I barely noticed, growing peacefully, perfectly… through all that spring excitement.

The rains that May were incredible, pouring and pouring for days – The green burst through, and flowers! I lay at night, listening to the downpour, and thought to myself that you were a girl, and that maybe your name would be "Iris Rain." I was so surprised at your coming! Your birthday seemed very far-off, though, and so I kept on planning and building our new little homestead, the wildfire in me still ablaze despite the rains.

Summer & Fall, 2015

By the end of May, I started to feel tired, and morning sickness slowed me down incredibly. The boundless energy I had felt in the spring was waning, and I found myself very irritable and stubborn – still determined to continue work on our homestead even though my body was slowing down.

The business of spring continued through summer, and I worked on all sorts of big and little projects with you inside me, and kept up with the garden. In July & August, we had so much to eat from our little farm that we didn't have to buy any vegetables or eggs from the store! And, although this work of growing our food was so physically and emotionally rewarding, I was exhausted.

Then, one night in September, I had a dream. It was fast and fiery, full of tension and movement. Then, the movement stopped, and remaining in its absence, clear and real, was FEAR. Fear of birth. Fear that my body would not be able to handle it this time… And in the midst of the fear, my own voice called out, as clear as clear could be, "HELP!" I woke immediately ~ completely lucid, completely clear… so surprised by what that dream had revealed.

Things had changed, and I was ignoring the change. Since I had had such a positive experience birthing Micah alone, I had been assuming that I would just to duplicate that birth… that it would be simple – easy – nothing to worry about – no planning necessary. But things had changed. You and I were calling, loud and clear, for support.

The Darkness Returns ~ October & November

That dream was a turning point in my pregnancy with you, sweet one. Things became dark, but not in a bad way – I needed that darkness – that inward movement. I needed the calm and the quiet. Things became slower, gentler... more organized and clear and soft. With the turning of the year towards the deep, dark winter, so my body turned.

I sat at night by candlelight, reading birth stories. I drank these birth stories in – they were nectar for my soul. I was suddenly SO excited to be connected with you, to birth you and care for you and be your mother.

I began to plan for your coming. I worried that Peacy and Micah would be distracting for me during labor, so I looked for a Doula, and found the perfect one. It was so good to have that reassurance – that safety net. If we needed to, we could call her to help with any of it - to watch the kids, or stoke the fires, or feed the goats & chickens....

In November, I met with a midwife. I was still unsure of why I was meeting with her, but it felt right somehow. When we met, I knew right away that I could trust her. She was patient and calm, completely accepting of my birth choices, completely accepting of everything I had to say. She didn't seem like a 'birth professional' – she was a wise woman who I could talk with openly. I told her my fears - what if something was to go wrong? Could there be trauma to the varicose veins around my yoni? What if Joey and I needed more help than a Doula could provide? What if the children were loud and distracting for me during birth?? It was so nice to talk with her, especially after rejecting midwifery care in my first two pregnancies. I began to see how amazing it could be to invite this woman into my life. She was a voice of wisdom and care, a true "sage femme," advocating for self-care and intuition.

Although I was still planning a freebirth, this midwife offered me her phone number, just in case I changed my mind last minute. I didn't need to sign a contract, make an agreement for payment, or make any agreement of any kind – she told me I could just call her if I wanted, as a friend in need rather than a 'client.' I felt so encouraged and blessed to have met with her! I felt like I had gotten a whole lot of baggage out of the way in one sitting, and now all that was left in front of me was the clear, free path to meeting you.

Waiting ~ December & January

I felt big and beautiful. I had found a routine, with my dark quiet nights, reading birth stories by the fire, candlelight showers after gentle days… I envisioned your ecstatic birth. I was so ready and excited to meet you!

Our home blossomed as I cleaned and arranged and made safe a place for your coming. Fires blazed in the woodstoves, and snow fell outside, and then more snow. I thought you would come on Solstice, but you waited.

We built a nursing bed by the woodstove in the middle room, and I envisioned you coming right there. I sewed and sewed every night – bedspreads, pillows, and lots and lots of new curtains to cover the windows. When I found myself sewing curtains, I really thought "you must be close!" When January came, I prepared each day for your coming, but you waited…

Our house really felt perfect – I had found such a good groove with keeping it clean and organized, and felt SO ready! Some nights I had what I thought might be contractions, and even the altered consciousness of birthing, but you waited, and I waited.

Then, around the beginning of January, we all got sick. Joey first, then Micah and Peacy, and then me… not just a little cold, but a real, big cold, with a raw, dry sore throat and a fever, congestion headaches and foggy exhaustion. I hadn't been that sick for a long time. Suddenly it hit me how cold it was outside. Going out to feed the goats, chickens & rabbits meant trudging through the snow, breaking the ice on their water buckets… and we had to bring in a whole wagon of wood each day to keep the fires hot enough to warm the house. Feeding the animals and keeping up with firewood seemed totally unmanageable. The house seemed to fall apart. The floors, which had been swept and tidy every day, were now strewn with snotty tissues, towels, dirty clothes, bits of kindling and wood dust… I made a big pot of chicken soup, and it was all that we ate for days. It all felt like too much, with the knowledge that you were so, so close to coming. I didn't feel like I had an ounce of energy left, not even enough to sweep the floor, let alone to give birth to you.

But after about a week, on the morning of January 15th, things lightened. Though the sore throat remained, some of my energy returned. I felt well enough again to make another big pot of chicken soup, and to thoroughly clean the kitchen and middle room. Peacy and Micah were still sick, but also feeling a bit better. They went to bed around nightfall. As I was tucking them into their blankets, I felt a stirring… I felt you. Deep down inside, I knew you were ready ~ you were coming.

The Night of your Birth

I said goodnight to Peacy and Micah, and turned off the bedroom lights. The house was quiet. Joey was up, on the computer. There were a few more dishes to do in the kitchen, and some more cleaning. As I was doing dishes, I felt you stir again… not a physical stirring, but something deeper – a calling out from you to me – a message. "Prepare, I am coming."

I almost smiled… was this really the night? After all this waiting, I really didn't expect it to be this night!

I kept on cleaning, and made some balls of honey mixed with slippery elm and rosehip powder. We'd been sucking on these all week to help with the sore throat.

You stirred again… this time, a contraction.

I felt so clear and alert… so aware. I completely forgot about

253

being sick.

A few minutes later, (maybe 10 minutes?), another contraction. This was the night!

I had to use the potty bucket a few times... all the while, so clear and present... so calm and ready. I was clearing my body for your passage.

I ran out of wood shavings for the potty bucket.

Joey came into the kitchen. I felt secretive... I felt interrupted... I didn't want to tell him what I knew was happening.

"We are going to need some more wood shavings for the potty bucket" I said.

"Now?" He obviously didn't want to get them, understandably; it was dark and cold outside where we had a bin of shavings in the woodshed.

"I need them tonight... I could get them if you don't want to... but..." I was so reluctant to say I was in labor, for some reason... maybe because I thought that saying it would make me a thing to observe, and I didn't want to be observed... but I said it anyways – "I think... I might be having contractions... I think the baby is coming tonight."

Once I had spoken about it, it became obvious that there was regularity and an increasing intensity to the contractions. It's amazing how vocalization can really solidify something like that...

Joey went to get wood shavings.

I started to get the house ready, and Joey helped. The last of the dishes were done. We put a basin of water on the woodstove, laid out towels, and brought the potty bucket into the middle room where I felt most comfortable. Fires were going in all of the stoves, and extra wood brought in. During this, some of the contractions were more intense, requiring more attention and movement.

Then Joey went to bed. The house was dark, save two candles, one of which was a beeswax rose candle that I had been saving for your birth, finally burning. Of course, just after Joey went to bed, things greatly intensified. Even after my realizations during pregnancy that I would benefit from support, I had still planned to birth you alone, just as I had with Micah. I was so thirsty, and drank a lot of water, and ate almost all of the slippery elm/honey balls that I had made (which were supposed to last for a few days, at least.) The tapered candle seemed too bright, so I blew it out, leaving just your rose candle burning. Things became very, very intense. I was on all fours in front of the woodstove, holding a warm cloth to my perineum, with olive oil. I felt like I had to pee, but every time I tried nothing came out. Back and forth, back and forth, from all fours to the potty bucket, with gulps of water in between... the energy so quick... my moans loud and low.... So, so intense... It became clear then, so clear, that your birth would not be as easy as Micah's. I called for help...

"Joey," I said quietly. And he came out of the bedroom, looking tired. Another contraction. "Can you bring me some orange juice, and some more water?" He brought it and placed it next to me by the middle room woodstove. I asked him to not to go back to bed – I asked him to stay with me.

With each contraction, I needed to hang onto the windowsill, pulling down and moaning loudly and deeply. I remember thinking right then, just after a contraction, "I will have to write this down, otherwise I will forget – I have to write down that this hurts, a lot!!" (Of course, now, I have forgotten – looking back it seems like it was blissful, and of course it was, but I am glad I noted in that moment, that there was real pain.) But there was no time then to write it down. There was only just enough time between contractions to rest for a few seconds.

I was grateful for Joey's presence. I knew he was there, but he wasn't obtrusive at all – just quiet and present.

I sat on the potty bucket, feeling like I needed to pee again, but unable to. The pressure felt unbearable. I reached up inside my yoni to see – to feel if you were close. I hadn't planned to check my progress at all, but this felt so instinctive, and not at all intrusive. I didn't feel you, and let my fingers slip out.

Another contraction came – it was painful. I rocked back and forth, moaning. And then another came, and then another! The feeling like I had to pee was really unbearable! I reached back up inside myself, instinctively again. I felt my cervix – it was barely there, stretchy and thin and almost gone. I felt the front wall of my yoni, and felt my bladder there, taking up too much space, full and hard. I pressed gently forwards on my bladder, and I was finally able to pee! And, just on the heels of that relief from finally being able to pee, there came a series of the most incredibly intense contractions! I was blown away, completely vulnerable as you opened me that last little bit. As those contractions came, without thought, I reached out to Joey and gestured in front of me, saying "I need you, right here!"

Joey came. I reached up to him and held onto his arms and pulled down, hard, with all of my weight and yours, through the contractions. He supported me under my armpits, and the relief from his support was instant. What felt like it would be impossible suddenly became so doable! I had something, someone, to pull against, to help you through me. I had found my support.

In between contractions, we let go of each other, but each time I felt another wave building, I called out, "again," and he was there. After a few times doing this, I could tell you had moved down. I reached inside myself again, just to see, and I felt you! Not too close, but there you were!

Those contractions while holding Joey were so effective, but they became so intense that I was desperate for some change! My body took me down quickly, onto my hands and knees on a mat in front of the woodstove, all despite my mind, which had chosen that time for a sudden uproar of, "Is this the right thing to do??? I don't know what to do!!" But I didn't need to heed that internal voice… it was fairly comical to hear the frantic inner commentary, but I paid no more attention to it than to notice it. I trusted my body. I felt such relief in that transition to hands & knees, for that is what it was… transition! You were on your way, descending.

Contraction after contraction, you were coming closer and closer.

My moans were so loud. I assumed I was waking up your brother and sister, but didn't know what else to do – the sound helped so much. I was on my knees, chest supported on the couch, my back end facing the woodstove, and in the middle of one of the most intense contractions, BURST!!

Waters!!!! They just exploded from behind me, like nothing I had ever felt before, for your sister and brother had been born with their waters. They barreled from me, so unexpectedly sudden! I felt SO open.. SO very vulnerable. I knew you must have been feeling the same way, suddenly exposed. My low moans turned to high-pitched, vulnerable gasps of air. I could feel the rush of hormones – the knowing that you were almost there – that I would be meeting so soon! You were coming! One or two more huge contractions, and I knew that in that intensity, I couldn't turn to catch you. "Come to catch!" I said to Joey.

He was there.

You were crowning, slowly, beautifully. I thought your head had passed through, but then to my surprise, it had only been the top of your head. Then I felt your little nose pop through, and then your little chin. It was a beautifully foreign feeling, how slowly and gracefully you came, especially after the turbulence of your labor.... Like the sun poking through the clouds after a particularly fierce thunderstorm. You rested for a moment, with your head outside of my body. Then I felt you, clearly, beautifully, gracefully turning inside of me. You paused again, and then you slid from me, into your fathers waiting hands, and then slipped down onto the mat. I turned and saw you, so tiny, like a little frog, belly down on a pile of wet towels. I will never forget that moment, beautiful Ahmik.

I picked you up and held you to my belly, fumbling. You were so slippery! Your breathing was raspy, full of mucous. I tried to clear it for you. I passed something big and wondered if it was your placenta, but realized it was just a bunch of large blood clots. Your cord was so short; I could barely reach you to my lap. I felt uncomfortable sitting, but unsteady and unsure of how to stand. I was shaking. Then your

placenta came, with more blood, and we decided you were ready –
your breathing was steady, and you had latched on – and we cut your
cord. You were there, a tiny being on your own for the first time, but
so safe and loved in my arms.

I stood, and more blood came. Joey helped me set up a little bed
on the couch for the night. I was so thirsty and hungry, and felt so
depleted. All of the feelings in my body, which had been outshined
by your coming, returned. I noticed how sore my throat still was.

Joey brought me lots of water and chocolate milk... he made me
more slippery elm honey, and got the fire going really well... and
then he went to bed. I lay there on the couch with you all night. You
seemed agitated. You latched on, but wouldn't suck for long periods,
and you cried a lot. Neither of us slept. I wanted to talk to you to
sooth you, but my throat felt so dry and scratchy and sore that I
couldn't. Then, dawn came – that first light after a long night, and I
found my voice – I sang to you... "sweet asela, sweet ah-sey-laa,
sweet asela, sweet ah-say-laa..." ... and your body relaxed, and you
fell asleep on my chest... like you had been waiting for my voice all
along. I fell asleep too.

I woke maybe an hour later to little voices coming from the
bedroom, interspersed with Joey's low voice. Your sister and brother
came out, beautiful as they always are in the mornings with ruffled
hair and newly shining eyes. They crawled into bed with us on the
couch, Joey standing nearby, looking at your little body in surprise.
We were all together – now a family of five.

Four days later, the sun warmed the earth enough to dig a hole.
We buried your placenta, and gave you your name.

Ahmik Ash Meadow Sunrise. Ash for the tree, strong and
graceful. Ahmik, meaning beaver, for family and home. Meadow for
your beautiful, verdant, interconnected soul, and Sunrise because you
are as bright and strong and clear as the morning sun. Your birthday
is January 15th, a Friday as I remember, just an hour or so before
midnight. As I write this, you are only four months old, but you have
brought so much joy to our family already!

The river is flowing, flowing and growing,

The river is flowing, down to the sea.

Oh mother carry me, your child I will always be,

Oh mother carry me, down to the sea ....

Resources & Suggested Reading

Pregnancy & Childbirth Books

* *Spiritual Midwifery* by Ina May Gaskin(Lots of beautiful birth stories from "The Farm" in Tennessee, plus insight into Ina May's training as a midwife. I would caution, however, that some information in this book seems outdated to me.)

* *The Sacred Nature of Birth* by Kara Maria Ananda (Beautifully written and spiritual in nature, with lots and lots of AMAZING birth stories at the end!)

* *Prenatal Yoga and Natural Birth* by Jeannine Parvati Baker (The best parts of this book are Jeannine's amazing childbirth stories. She writes with a lightness and sense of humor while conveying the amazing power of childbirth. The beginning of the book is dedicated to her yoga practices, which are nice if you like yoga.)

* *The Birthkeepers* by Veronika Sophia Robinson (One of my greatest inspirations – Veronika's book is very opinionated but beautiful, and the birth stories at the end are the best I have ever read.)

* *Birth Unhindered* by Tara L. McGuire (Details of Tara's amazing pregnancy and birth journeies.)

* *Heart & Hands* by Elizabeth Davis (A practical guide for midwives.)

* *Gentle Birth, Gentle Mothering* by Sarah Buckley (Evidence-based information on natural childbirth and care of infants.)

* *The Natural Pregnancy Book* by Aviva Jill Romm (A great resource, especially the last section on home remedies during pregnancy.)

* *Wise Woman Herbal for the Childbearing Year* by Susun Weed (My copy is so worn that the pages are falling out!)

Parenting Books

* *The Continuum Concept* by Jean Leidloff (An examination of the contrast between modern American child-raising in a nuclear family and the ancient child-raising practices of an Amazonian tribe.)

* *How To Talk So Kids Will Listen & Listen So Kids Will Talk* by Adele Faber & Elaine Mazlish (Helpful communication skills for parents.)

* *Raising Our Children, Raising Ourselves* by Naomi Aldort (Absolutely the best parenting book I have ever read!)

* *Everyday Blessings: The Inner Work of Mindful Parenting* by Myla & Jon Kabat-Zinn (Great insight into the inner work of parents striving for a meaningful, respectful relationship with their children.)

* *Siblings Without Rivalry* by Adele Faber & Elaine Mazlish (An indispensable resource for parents with multiple children. Read it *before* they get old enough to start fighting!)

* *Naturally Healthy Babies & Children* by Aviva Jill Romm (An amazing resource – simple home health care for kids of all ages.)

* *Nonviolent Communication* by Marshall B. Rosenberg (Not specific to parenting, but one of the most useful relationship tools I have come across thus far. It is highly applicable to parenting.)

* *Healing Stories for Challenging Behavior* by Susun Perrow (An amazing resource for parents – we can become amazing storytellers and in doing so, can nourish the imaginative and creative hearts of our children.)

* *Welcoming Spirit Home* by Sobonfu Some (A beautiful look at the essential rituals of Sobonfu's village in Africa – rituals which relate to relationship, pregnancy, childbirth, and children.)

Websites

* *Stand & Deliver* – Plenty of evidence-based information on pregnancy and childbirth, including free PDF downloads of Rixa's PhD dissertation "Born Free: Unassisted Childbirth in North America" and other publications. (rixarixa.blogspot.com)

* *Center for Unhindered Living's online childbirth class* – A site dedicated to unhindered living! This (free) class focuses on taking control of your birth experience and having a truly unhindered birth.(www.unhindered-living.com/the-online-childbirth-class.html)

* *IndieBirth* – "offers concrete knowledge, ancient wisdom and current research [to pregnant women and midwives] so women can make choices with full awareness, from the full spectrum of choices." Excellent podcasts!(www.indiebirth.com)

* *Birth Without Fear Blog* –Loads of amazing birth stories, from unassisted to hospital birth, with photos, videos, etc. (birthwithoutfearblog.com)

* *Spinning Babies* – Fetal positioning, belly mapping, birth anatomy, techniques to ease difficult labors, birth stories and more! (www.spinningbabies.com)

Are you looking for more stories of unhindered childbirth?

I'm working on compiling a new book, solely dedicated to unhindered birth stories. If you'd like to get a free digital copy of the book once it's available, sign up by sending your first name and email address to sarah.m.haydock@gmail.com, and you'll be added to the list of recipients!

Want to share your story?

Your story could be so inspirational for those who are just embarking on the journey of freebirth! If you are interested in contributing your story to my new book, send me an email and we can get started: sarah.m.haydock@gmail.com

References

A.M. Jukic, D.D. Baird, C.R. Weinberg, D.R. McConnaughey and A.J. Wilcox. (2013) *Length of human pregnancy and contributors to its natural variation.* Oxford Journals. http://humrep.oxfordjournals.org/content/early/2013/08/06/humrep.det297.full

Azuzay Zamani. (2001) *Traditional Practices in Postnatal Care: The Malay Community In Malaysia,* TSMJ Volume 2

Boyda-Vikander, Svea. (2012) *Mothering the Mother: 40 Days of Rest.* Birth Without Fear Blog. http://birthwithoutfearblog.com/2012/10/21/mothering-the-mother-40-days-of-rest/

Braconnier, Deborah (April 21, 2011) *Chimpanzee birth similar to humans: study.* http://phys.org/news/2011-04-chimpanzee-birth-similar-humans.html

Buckley, Sarah J. (2009) *Gentle Birth, Gentle Mothering: A Doctor's Guide to Natural Childbirth and Gentle Early Parenting Choices.* Celestial Arts

Buckley, Sarah J. (2005) *Hormones in Labour and Birth – How your body helps you.* www.bellybelly.com.au/birth/ecstatic-birth-natures-hormonal-blueprint-for-labor

Buhner, Stephen H. (2004) *The Secret Teachings of Plants: the intelligence if the heart in the direct perception of nature.* Rochester, VT: Bear & Company

Clark, Demetria. *What Herbs Are Good for Labor?* Midwives Herbal, Part Two. http://birtharts.com/HerbsforLabor.pdf

Colson, Suzanne. (2012) *Biological Nurturing: The Laid-back Breastfeeding Revolution.* Midwifery Today. http://www.midwiferytoday.com/articles/biologicalnurturing.asp

Condon,Jennifer C., Jeyasuria,Pancharatnam, Faust,Julie M., and Mendelson, Carole R. *Surfactant protein secreted by the maturing mouse fetal lung acts as a hormone that signals the initiation of parturition.* PNAS, vol. 101 no. 14. (2004.) http://www.pnas.org/content/101/14/4978.full?sid=addd2e9b-c5dc-49e7-9074-2480bad272fa

Dettwyler, Katherine A. (2011) *Cultural Anthropology & Human Experience.* Waveland Press, Inc.

Edwards, Gail Faith. (2000) *Opening Our Wild Hearts to the Healing Herbs.* Woodstock NY: Ash Tree Publishing

Fetal Lungs Protein Release Triggers Labor to Begin. Peaceful Parenting. (2010) http://www.drmomma.org/2008/01/fetal-lungs-protein-release-triggers.html

Fox, Harold. *Aging of the placenta.* ADC, Fetal and Neonatal Edition.

(1997.) http://fn.bmj.com/content/77/3/F171.full

Gaskin, Ina May. (1975) *Spiritual Midwifery*. Summertown, TN: Book Publishing Company

Gladstar, Rosemary. (2001) *Herbal Recipes for Vibrant Health*. North Adams, MA: Storey Publishing

Goer, Henci. *Gestational Diabetes: The Emperor as No Clothes*. The Birth Gazette, Spring 1996, Vol.12 No. 2. http://www.gentlebirth.org/archives/gdhgoer.html

Hardin, Kiva Rose. *10 Reasons to Love Motherwort*. http://bearmedicineherbals.com/10-reasons-to-love-motherwort.html

Hart, Gail. *A Timely Birth*. Midwifery Today, Issue 72. (Winter 2004.) https://www.midwiferytoday.com/articles/timely.asp

Hirata, Satoshi. Fuwa, Koki, Sugama, Keiko. Kusunoki, Kiyo & Takeshita, Hideko. (April 20, 2011) *Mechanism of birth in chimpanzees: humans are not unique among primates*. Royal Society Publishing. http://rsbl.royalsocietypublishing.org/content/7/5/686.full

Jukic AM, Baird DD, Weinberg CR, McConnaughey DR, Wilcox AJ. *Length of human pregnancy and contributors to its natural variation*. (2013) http://www.ncbi.nlm.nih.gov/pubmed/23922246

Kaminski, Patricia & Katz, Richard. (1986) *Flower Essence Reparatory*. Nevada City, CA: Flower Essence Society

Kendall-Tackett, Kathleen. (2011) *How Other Cultures Prevent Postpartum Depression*. Kindred Community.

http://www.kindredcommunity.com/2011/10/how-other-cultures-prevent-postpartum-depression/

Kresser, Chris. *Natural childbirth: the evolutionary template for birth.* http://chriskresser.com/naturalchildbirth

Leboyer, Frederick. (2006) *The Art of Giving Birth.* Rochester, VT: Healing Arts Press

Littlejohn, Marrianne. (2011) *Birth in South Africa: Indigenous Traditions.* Spiritual Birth. http://www.spiritualbirth.net/birth-in-south-africa-indigenous-traditions

Mongon, Marie. (1992) *Hypnobirthing: The Mongan Method.* Deerfield Beach, FL: Health Communications, Inc.

Pitman, Theresa. (2003) *Infant Self Attachment.* LEAVEN, Vol. 38 No. 6, December 2002 - January 2003, pp. 123-125. La Leche League, International. http://www.llli.org/llleaderweb/lv/lvdecjan03p123.html

Ptak G E, Tacconi E, Czernik M, Toschi P, Modlinski JA, Loi P.*Embryonic diapause is conserved across mammals.* (2012.) http://www.ncbi.nlm.nih.gov/pubmed/22427933

Ptak G E, Modlinski J A,Loi P.*Embryonic diapause in humans: time to consider?.* (2013) http://www.ncbi.nlm.nih.gov/pmc/articles/PMC3848826/

Robinson, Veronika Sophia. (2008) *The Birthkeepers: Reclaiming an Ancient Tradition.* Starflower Press

Romm, Aviva Jill. (1997) *The Natural Pregnancy Book.* New York: Celestial Arts

Spinning Babies. (2012-2013) Maternity House Publishing, Inc. http://spinningbabies.com

Some, Sobonfu E. (1999) *Welcoming Spirit Home: Ancient African Teachings to Celebrate Children & Community.* Novato CA: New World Library.

Weed, Susun S. (1986) *Wise Woman Herbal for the Childbearing Year.* Woodstock, NY: Ash Tree Publishing

Wood, Matthew. (1997) The Book of Herbal Wisdom: using plants as medicines. Berkley, CA: North Atlantic Books